Gastric Sleeve Cookbook

The Ultimate Guide To Eating Healthy Pre And Post-Op Gastric Sleeve with Delicious Recipes

By

Angela Ramsey

© **Copyright 2022 by Angela Ramey- All rights reserved.**

This document is geared towards providing exact and reliable information regarding the topic and issue covered.

- From a Declaration of Principles, which was accepted and approved equally by a Committee of the American Bar Association and a Committee of Publishers and Associations.

It is not legal to reproduce, duplicate, or transmit any part of this document in either electronic means or printed format. All rights reserved.

The information provided herein is stated to be truthful and consistent. Any liability, in terms of inattention or otherwise, by any usage or abuse of any policies, processes, or directions contained within is the sole responsibility of the recipient reader. Under no circumstances will any legal obligation or blame be held against the publisher for any reparation, damages, or monetary loss due to the information herein, either directly or indirectly.

Respective authors own all copyrights not held by the publisher.

The information herein is solely offered for informational purposes and is universal. The presentation of the data is without a contract or any guaranteed assurance.

The trademarks used are without any consent, and the trademark publication is without permission or backing by the trademark owner. All trademarks and brands within this book are for clarifying purposes only, owned by themselves, and not affiliated with this document.

Contents

INTRODUCTION 6

CHAPTER 1: INTRODUCTION TO GASTRIC SLEEVE 7

    1.1: What is a Gastric Sleeve? 7

    1.2: Pre-Op Gastric Sleeve Diet 8

CHAPTER 2: POST-OPERATION FOODS 11

    2.1: Week 1 11

    2.2: Week 2 12

    2.3: Week 3 13

    2.4: Week 4 13

    2.5: Week 5 14

CHAPTER 3: BREAKFAST RECIPES 17

    3.1: Plain Frittata with Eggs 17

    3.2: High Protein Pancakes 19

    3.3: Cheddar Zucchini Muffins 20

    3.4: Hawaiian Hash 21

    3.5: Mushroom Breakfast Burritos 22

    3.6: Cinnamon Apples 24

    3.7: Chia Blueberry Oats 25

    3.8: Avocado Toast with Boiled Eggs 26

    3.9: Creamy Oatmeal Porridge 27

    3.10: Blueberry Almond Porridge 28

CHAPTER 4: SNACKS AND SIDES 29

    4.1: Chia Seed Pudding 29

    4.2: Pumpkin Muffins 30

    4.3: Keto Soft Pretzels 31

    4.4: Spinach Artichoke Dip 33

    4.5: Chocolate Peanut Butter Bites 35

    4.6: Cinnamon Apple Porridge 37

    4.7: Tuna Salad Stuffed Tomatoes 38

    4.8: Turkey, Avocado, and Cheddar Wrap 39

    4.9: Shrimp Kabobs 40

    4.10: Grilled Chicken with Vegetables 41

INVITE TO REVIEW BOOK 42

CHAPTER 5: LUNCH RECIPES 43

5.1: High-Protein Chicken Soup 43

5.2: Baked Ricotta 44

5.3: Butterfly Chicken 46

5.4: Vegetable Khichdi 48

5.5: Tuna Sandwich 500

5.6: Whole-wheat Broccoli Pasta 51

5.7: Keto Enchidilas 53

5.8: White Chicken 55

CHAPTER 6: DESSERT AND SMOOTHIE RECIPES 56

6.1: Blueberry Cupcakes Lemon Icing 56

6.2: Carrot Cake 58

6.3: Apple Chunks Oatmeal Cookies 59

6.4: Chocolate Cake 61

6.5: Pear and Ginger smoothie 63

6.6: Mixed Berry Smoothie 64

6.7: Orange Smoothie 66

6.8: Dragon Fruit Smoothie 67

6.9: Peanut Butter Banana Porridge 68

6.10: Creamy Rice Porridge 69

CHAPTER 7: DINNER RECIPES 70

7.1: Meatloaf Muffins with Barbecue 70

7.2: Chicken Fajita Bowls 72

7.3: Garlic Butter Salmon 74

7.4: Cauliflower Casserole 75

7.5: Bell Pepper Soup 77

7.6: Chickpea Curry 79

7.7: Mushroom Sauce Meatloaf 81

7.8: Pressure Cooker Apple Chicken 83

7.9: Baked Salmon with Roasted Broccoli 85

7.10: Turkey Chili 86

CHAPTER 8: SOUPS AND STEWS RECIPES 87

8.1: Tummy Healing Soup 87

- 8.2: Onion Thyme Soup 88
- 8.3: Broccoli and Sweet Potato Soup 90
- 8.4: Cabbage Stew 92
- 8.5: Chicken Soup Stew 94
- 8.6: Harvest Soup 96
- 8.7: Spicy Bean Soup 97
- 8.8: Healing Vegetable Soup 98
- 8.9: Veggie Lentil Soup 99
- 8.10: Grilled Chicken Broth Bowl 100

CHAPTER 9: PUREE RECIPES 101
- 9.1: Sweet Salmon Puree 101
- 9.2: Avocado Puree 102
- 9.3: Mango and Peanut Butter Puree 103
- 9.4: Vegetable Soup Puree 104
- 9.5: Pumpkin Puree 105
- 9.6: Mix Vegetable Puree 106

CHAPTER 10: TIPS FOR DINING OUT 107
- 10.1: When will you be able to begin eating out? 108
- 10.2: What Food Should One Eat? 109
- 10.3: Take Control when Selecting Beverage 109
- 10.4: Better Choices From Different Restaurants 110
- 10.5: Extra Tips 111

CONCLUSION 113

INVITE TO REVIEW BOOK 114

Introduction

One of the most common bariatric procedures nowadays is "Sleeve Gastrostomy"; "vertical sleeve gastrostomy" is also used. Laparoscopic surgery is often used for this operation, which entails introducing tiny tools via several tiny incisions in the upper belly. The stomach is removed from the body, leaving behind a tube-shaped stomach about the shape and size of a banana.

After having bariatric surgery, it might not be easy to reevaluate and alter your previous eating patterns. Thanks to the availability of bariatric cookbooks, patients may find nourishing foods that are also healthful and rich in protein. You can create the route that leads to a proper post-op diet with the help of the appropriate bariatric cookbook. Consuming meals high in protein is vital for people who have had bariatric procedures like gastric sleeve. No added sugar is in any recipes, and most do not include gluten. This cookbook offers a broad range of tastes by providing recipes for many cuisines that are easy to prepare and do not need much time. Some cuisines include French, Italian, Indian, and Caribbean foods.

This book is much more than a simple cookbook. It suggests adopting appropriate portion sizes and increasing the amount of protein in the meals. A more thorough comprehension of typical serving sizes will eliminate the need for bariatric portion control plates. These meals should be easy to include in your bariatric diet and food list for gastric bypass surgery. It will proceed in tandem with the stages of your eating. The dishes are mouthwatering no matter what form they take—whether they are solid, mashed, or diced. This book provides an overview of meals you can consume, such as complete liquids, vegetarian meals, soft foods, protein drinks, especially for bariatric patients, slow cooker dinners, and almost a hundred more nutritious and tasty dishes. In the cookbook, different recovery stages are represented by different icons, so you can easily choose the meals that are most suited to your current state.

Chapter 1: Introduction to Gastric Sleeve

The gastric sleeve, commonly known as sleeve gastrostomy, is an operation performed during bariatric surgery to cause the patient to lose weight. Your stomach will get smaller due to using it, which is how it works. The surgical removal of all or part of a person's stomach is called a "gastrostomy." The gastric sleeve procedure involves removing around 80% of the stomach and replacing it with a tube-like "sleeve" comparable in size and shape to a banana.

1.1: What is a Gastric Sleeve?

It is possible to reduce the quantity of food consumed in a single sitting by decreasing the size of the stomach, which will also cause you to feel fuller more quickly. However, it also accomplishes another goal: to lessen the quantity of appetite your stomach can create. This helps to suppress both your appetite and cravings, and it also has the potential to block the impulses that lead individuals to gain back the weight they've reduced.

How frequent is gastric sleeve procedure?

The gastric sleeve procedure is the kind of weight reduction surgery that is done the most often both in the United States and throughout the globe. In the United States, sleeve gastrostomies account for more than half of all weight loss procedures carried out annually. Around 150,000 gastric sleeve surgeries are done annually in the United States, and 380,000 are performed annually throughout the globe. However, just 1% of those who potentially benefit from the operation and who meet the requirements to have it get it.

Which medical issues may be treated with the help of gastric sleeve surgery?

Surgical therapy for obesity and the medical issues associated with obesity may take the form of gastric sleeve surgery. It is only made available to persons who qualify for it, and either already have major medical disorders due to their obesity or are at a high risk of acquiring such diseases. Gastric sleeve surgery has the potential to treat, and in some cases even cure, a variety of disorders, including but not limited to:

- Insulin resistance and diabetes type 2 are synonymous terms.
- Hypertension, as well as cardiac disease caused by hypertension.

- High blood fat levels, and hyperlipidemia, are linked to artery disease.
- Steatohepatitis and nonalcoholic fatty liver cancer go hand in hand.
- Both obesity, cerebral hypoxia syndrome, and disruptive sleep apnea are associated with obesity.
- Symptoms of osteoarthritis include joint discomfort.

Is gastric sleeve a risk-free procedure?

The hazards of being overweight and the associated illnesses are far higher than the risks of undergoing gastric sleeve surgery. It also has reduced rates of complications compared to other popular surgeries, such as gallbladder removal and hip replacement. Most gastric sleeve surgeries are carried out using minimally invasive surgical methods. This results in reduced discomfort due to the incisions and a quicker recovery time.

1.2: Pre-Op Gastric Sleeve Diet

Your eating routine in the time leading up to your gastric sleeve surgery will follow the guidelines in the pre-op diet. Your eating habits are very important to the outcome of the operation for three reasons:

- It makes the treatment simpler to do while also making it safer. The pre-op diet is designed to reduce the amount of fat accumulated around the liver, making it easier for the surgeon to reach the stomach.
- It lessens the likelihood of experiencing difficulties. Losing weight may reduce the likelihood of experiencing adverse health effects before and after surgical procedures, which are made more likely by obesity.
- It gets you started on the behaviors necessary to maintain a lifetime commitment to maintaining a healthy weight. You'll get assurance from planning your future and completing it.
- When preparing for a bariatric operation, your pre-op diet should typically begin three weeks before the scheduled surgery. For more information on when you should start your diet, please see the dietitian or coordinator of the program you are participating in.

3 Weeks Before Surgery

During the three weeks leading up to your operation, you will often arrange your meals such that they:

- Cut down on calories, particularly carbs. The majority of the calories that are consumed in the diets of Americans come from carbohydrates. It is recommended that refined sugars, such as those found in confectionery and soft drinks, be avoided. Other carbs, such as bread and pasta, aren't inherently unhealthy, but restricting how much of them you eat may benefit your weight management efforts.
- Maximize protein consumption. Consume at least sixty grams of protein daily. Salmon, eggs, poultry, and ground beef with a low-fat content all provide excellent protein sources.
- Pay attention to the beneficial fats. The idea that all fat is unhealthy for you is just a misconception. Some are, and some aren't. Foods such as fish, almonds, and olives are examples of foods that contain healthy fats. Other fats, such as those found in margarine or oils, need to have their consumption reduced. Complete avoidance of trans fats is strongly recommended.
- Don't dehydrate. In the weeks following your surgery, drink lots of water. Cut down on or eliminate your intake of soft drinks or alcoholic drinks.
- It is recommended by many weight loss programs that individuals consume between 800 and 1,200 calories per day and continue to adhere to these dietary requirements up until two to three days before their gastric sleeve surgical operation. To get more information, kindly see your program coordinator or dietitian.

Two to Three Days Before the Procedure

You must transition to a diet consisting mostly of liquids two to three days before your procedure. Limit your consumption of meals to liquids such as water, broth, hydrocolloids, and low-calorie carbonated beverages (no sodas). Beginning at noon on the day of your operation, you must refrain from consuming anything, even water. If you do not adhere to these requirements, you risk having your eligibility again for gastric sleeve treatment called into question.

What Should Be Done About Medication?

In addition, several drugs require that you stop using them before surgery. Among them are:

- Medicines for the treatment of arthritis
- NSAIDs include aspirin and other medications similar to aspirin, including Tylenol, Advil, Motrin, or Aleve.
- Herbal supplements
- Medications that thin the blood are often known as anticoagulants.

If you have questions or concerns about the limitations placed on your medicine before surgery, consult your primary care physician.

Chapter 2: Post-Operation Foods

Suppose you are considering getting a gastric sleeve operation. In that case, you are probably excited about your new body and the prospect of learning to eat in an entirely different manner. Exciting and taxing simultaneously, getting ready for life following a gastric sleeve operation will be an adventure for you. The diet you will be required to observe before and after the operation is highly particular and oriented toward assisting in recovery and preventing complications. As time goes on, your diet will become more focused on teaching you how to develop healthy eating habits. This will allow you to continue your weight loss journey and, ultimately, to maintain a healthy body weight for the rest of your life. We advise patients to only consume liquids for the first week after having a gastric sleeve, such as water, Crystal Light, sweetened tea with a little bit of Splenda, Powerade zero, and other minimal sugar drinks.

We will likely begin including protein drinks into your diet during the first week. You can add some protein to your diet with these shakes, which are high in protein, and nutrients and low in calories. Adding protein to your diet can assist with the recovery process.

2.1: Week 1

It would help if you stuck to the same diet of clear liquids you had consumed in the days preceding the operation for one week after the treatment was complete. This can be avoided by preventing postoperative problems such as intestinal blockage, gastric leakage, diarrhea, constipation, and dehydration. Your body requires rest to heal; following this routine will help you achieve that objective. Some things should keep in mind. Be careful to drink a lot of liquids that are clear in color. If you are having difficulties staying hydrated, you should consult your physician about the possibility of trying out some electrolyte beverages, such as Gatorade, that are low in calories. Avoid drinking anything that contains sugar. Sugar can factor in dumping syndrome when the small intestine quickly absorbs excessive sugar. These effects include extreme nausea, tiredness, diarrhea, and sometimes vomiting.

Additionally, sugar is an empty-calorie food source. It is best to abstain from doing so and cut back as much as possible in the long run. Caffeine, linked to both acid reflux & dehydration, is another substance that should be avoided. There is a correlation between drinking carbonated beverages, such as those containing sugar, those with no-calorie choices, and seltzer and experiencing bloating and gas. All of these should be avoided in the postoperative period and maybe even for the rest of your life.

After having bariatric surgery, maintaining adequate hydration will be the most critical thing you can do for your diet. Be sure to drink clear liquids (drinks higher in calories and protein) between meals. Take small sips and cease when you feel any pressure or fullness in your stomach. Dietitians typically recommend beginning with 200 milliliters (ml) per hour and gradually increasing this amount as tolerated. Aim to consume between 1.5 and 2 liters of water per day. Within a week of having surgery, you should make it a priority to eat at least 60 grams of protein per day. This is equivalent to drinking three pints of nutritious liquids such as milk or low-calorie drinks and an additional pint of clear fluid like water or squash. Getting enough protein daily can help your body heal from surgery and make it easier to maintain muscle mass while cutting calories and reducing overall body fat. In addition to the antacid medication recommended for you, such as lansoprazole, you should also take a completely chewable A-Z multivitamin throughout this period.

2.2: Week 2

You will transition to a diet consisting entirely of liquids during the third week after surgery. Nutrition shakes without sugar, such as Ensure Light instant breakfast drinks shakes manufactured with protein powder and other similar products. Thin soup and cream-based soups without lumps are acceptable; very modest soft soup noodles are recommended. Unsweetened milk and pudding that is low in sugar and fat-free frozen yogurt, desserts, and sorbet that is low in sugar and fat-free plain Greek yogurt that is fat-free fruit juices that do not contain pulp that has been diluted with hot water cereals that are thinned with water such as Lotion of Wheat or oatmeal. During this time, you could find a greater desire to eat. That is very normal, but it hardly justifies eating solid meals. Your stomach continues to struggle to process solids.

You may end up throwing up, along with additional issues. You can better prepare yourself for the next phase of your diet by drinking enough liquids and avoiding foods high in sugar and fat. Caffeine and carbonated beverages are still things you should stay away from. At this point, the food must be pulverized, crushed, or otherwise processed into a texture comparable to that of baby food. Aim to consume just moderately sized meals—five to Six times a day, with three main meals and two to three snacks in between. A portion of food is equal to between five and six tablespoons, or around a half cup to a cup. First, one should consume foods high in protein, following veggies, and finally, consuming fruits or carbohydrates. During this period, you may still require one to two quarts of nutrient-rich fluid (such as milk) to meet your daily protein requirements of sixty grams. You should eat your meal slowly, eating bites no bigger than a twenty-pound piece, and chew your food very thoroughly. Because your digestive system may be sensitive to spicy foods, you should consider incorporating them into your diet gradually and in limited quantities. Maintain a steady intake of fluids throughout the day, but avoid drinking with your meals for the time being. Before and after eating, you should hold off on drinking anything for half an hour. Drinking while you eat will make you feel full much more quickly, which may make you bloated, throw you up, and reduce your nourishment. The nutritionist you work with will provide an example of a food plan to follow.

2.3: Week 3

In the third week of the diet, you can eat pureed or very soft meals. Eating gently and thoroughly chewing your food, ideally at least 20-25 times before swallowing, is essential. It is allowed to consume any food that is low in fat, does not include any sugar, and can be pureed. This includes lean food sources and veggies that are not fibrous. It would help if you initiated an increase in the amount of protein you consume. Continue to consume eggs daily or drink sugar-free protein shakes if the taste of mashed lean protein sources is not to your liking. These kinds of foods can be consumed in infant food stored in jars, and Tofu made from silk that has been cooked, pureed white fish, eggs scrambled or soft-boiled, soup, cottage cheese, and fruit packed in juice in cans. Bananas that have been mashed, ripe mango blended into hummus, or mashed avocado, Greek yogurt in its purest form. Maintain your abstinence from coffee and chunky or solid foods throughout this time. You should also eat food that is unseasoned or has minimal seasoning if at all possible. It's possible that spices are to blame for your heartburn.

2.4: Week 4

You are now at the point one month after surgery where you can gradually reintroduce solid foods into your diet. Now is the occasion to put your newly acquired knowledge about healthy eating into practice and to do so with full vigor. Foods that are hard to absorb, such as steak, starchy vegetables, and nuts, should still be avoided. Alcohol and fat, particularly high-fat dairy products, should still be avoided. It would help if one steered precise pasta, white potatoes, and other high-carb alternatives. It is usually OK to begin consuming caffeinated beverages again now, provided that moderation is practiced. The following foods could be added to your list: chicken and fish that have been properly cooked, vegetables that have been cooked to a proper texture, sweet potatoes and cheese with a lower fat content fruit cereal with less sugar. It would be best to consume mushy or mashed foods about six to seven weeks after having bariatric surgery. The consistency of shepherd's pie or dhal should be your goal. You can try minced beef, fish, and chicken; hummus; scrambled eggs; cereals; cooked vegetables; canned fruits; and rice pudding (no added sugar). Try to stay away from foods that are heavy in fat and sugar.

Aim to eat three square meals and some nutritious snacks each day. Continue trying out your body with one different food each time so you can gauge how it reacts to various foods. Always remember to drink lots of fluids each day, nearly every day, but avoid doing so when you are eating. You may still require one pint of a nutrient-rich drink such as milk to meet your daily protein requirements of sixty grams. As soon as you feel you have a handle on soft meals, it would help to introduce crisp things, such as crackers, bread sticks, crispbread, and crispy toast. Stay away from anything that has a doughy consistency, like bread or chapattis, as these are nevertheless likely to give you some issues. At this stage, you can also introduce the "warning foods" discussed earlier in the process gradually.

2.5: Week 5

It is time to put the new standard eating plan into long-term effect now that you can consume solid food without risking your health. Maintain a diet high in lean protein and veggies, and when adding new foods to your diet, do it one at a time to gauge how your body reacts to each new item. Sugary candies and soda are foods you should either abstain entirely from in the future or consume only on rare occasions. Every other food can be reintroduced as long as it is not the food that causes the symptoms. Make informed decisions about the foods you eat by selecting options high in nutrients and avoiding meals low in these nutrients. You might find it easier to adhere to your diet if you divide each meal into three smaller portions and limit the snacks you consume. In extra to that, make sure that you are always well-hydrated. The following are some postoperative rehabilitation recommendations that can assist you in maintaining your routine. To puree food, you can use a blending or a food processor; to determine how to differentiate between the bodily sensation of hunger and the mental and emotional state of appetite. Avoid overeating because your stomach will get more elastic over time and eventually reach a stable size. Take your time when chewing and eating, Avoid non-nutrient calories, and steer clear of sweets in concentrated forms.

To avoid nutrient deficiency, you must take the following dietary supplements daily. Please remember that any pills must be broken up into bits no more significant than six to eight millimeters. You cannot absorb whole tablets as well as before the operation, and it may be challenging for the tablets to pass past your newly altered anatomy. Multivitamins Consume one serving of a high-potency chewable vitamin & mineral supplement daily. After your surgery, you should take two tablets every day for at least three months and one tablet every day for the rest of your life. Calcium Supplement Calcium intake should range from 1,200 mg to 2,000 mg daily to protect against nutritional deficiencies and bone damage. Calcium should be consumed in two to three staggered dosages throughout the day for optimal absorption. For instance, a supplement ranging from 500 to 600 milligrams should be consumed thrice daily.

The type of calcium that is most commonly used is calcium citrate. Vitamin D Supplement Vitamin D should be consumed in 800 to 6 thousand units (IUs) daily. This entire quantity should be consumed twice daily in 400 to 500 international units. Your calcium supplement should be used with vitamin D. If you would instead not take numerous tablets, you can choose to take a supplement that combines calcium and vitamin D, provided that it includes the appropriate amounts. Vitamin B12 Supplement Every day, you should take 500 mg of vitamin B. Tablets or sublingual versions inserted under the tongue are both acceptable administration methods. Additional Supplements Some patients, particularly women who continue to have menstruation, require supplementary folic acid and iron supplements. These patients can be identified by their lack of periods. This is something that your nutritionist will talk to you about.

Steer clear of fried, processed, and quick foods and trans fats. Drinking water or reduced-calorie versions of Gatorade can help you avoid becoming dehydrated. It's best to avoid eating and drinking at the same time. Discuss with your primary care physician the bariatric nutrients and supplements available to determine what to take and when you should take them. Integrate physical activity into your daily routine. The walk is a great place to start, and then you can branch out into other activities like swimming, dancing, and yoga. Avoid alcohol. Gastric sleeve operations and other bariatric operations may hasten and intensify the effects of drinking. Ibuprofen, aspirin, and naproxen are nonsteroidal anti-inflammatory medications (NSAIDs) that should be avoided. These common well-over pain medications can thin the natural layer protecting your stomach.

Chapter 3: Breakfast Recipes

3.1: Plain Frittata with Eggs

Prep Time: 20 minutes

Cook Time: 10 minutes

Servings: 1

Difficulty level: Easy

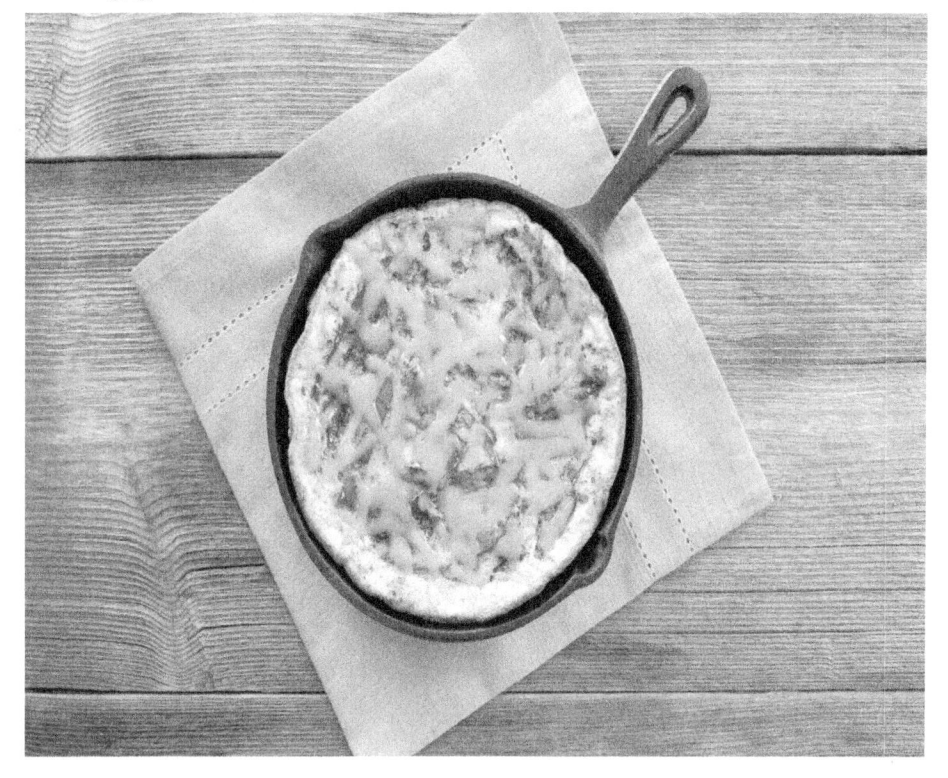

Ingredients

2 tablespoons chopped green bell pepper	½ ripe plantain
1 small size potato	¼ teaspoon onion powder
1 tablespoon green onion	a pinch of dry thyme
1 egg	¼ teaspoon salt or less
1/8 teaspoon black pepper	¼ teaspoon vegetable bullion or ¼ cube
1 clove of garlic, grated	¼ head of broccoli
1/4 small/medium size onion bulb	1/8 teaspoon crushed red pepper
1 teaspoon olive oil	2 teaspoon red bell pepper

Instructions

1. After following the instructions for washing and cutting the veggies, put them to the side. The potatoes are first precooked in water, brought to a boil after being rinsed and then sliced into pieces measuring 12 inches. The water is allowed to drain.

2. Start preparing the plantain by bringing a frying pan to a high temperature on the stove. After the plantain has been cut and a little coating of salt applied, the frying process may begin as soon as the oil has reached the desired temperature. Fry the plantain on all sides, and as soon as it is done, remove it from the oil and place it on a plate lined with paper towels. Continue cooking the plantains until they are finished, at which point, set them aside. After allowing the hot oil to cool down, gently pour it out of the container. The next step is to give the potatoes a quick sauté in the same pan; this step is entirely discretionary, but it brings out the full flavor of the potatoes.

3. Place a sanitized pot or pan on the heating element.

4. Warm up a half tablespoon of fresh olive oil in a skillet, add a bit of salt, and then add one cup of coarsely diced onions to the pan. Allow the onions to cook until they are translucent. After around three minutes, the broccoli may be added to the pan. After that, add the additional components, whisk, and mix everything until it is completely incorporated. After that, taste to check for tastes and adjust as necessary. Don't overcook these veggies; remember that they will still need to be baked later. Turn the stove off by moving the knob to the "off" position.

5. After they have been sautéed, transfer the veggies to a clean tray and set them aside for a while so that they may cool down.

6. While the oven is preheated at 350 degrees, you should have a baking pan ready and set aside. After that, break all ten eggs into a big bowl, add salt, pepper, and a few drops of vegetable bouillon, and then mix the ingredients. Then, gradually stir in the ingredients already sautéed in the previous step. Bake for thirty to forty minutes until the center of the dish can be tested with a toothpick and found clean.

| **Nutrition Facts** | Calories: 359 calories, Proteins: 32g, Carbs:16 g, Fat: 7g |

3.2: High Protein Pancakes

Prep Time: 3 minutes

Cook Time: 5 minutes

Servings: 1

Difficulty level: Easy

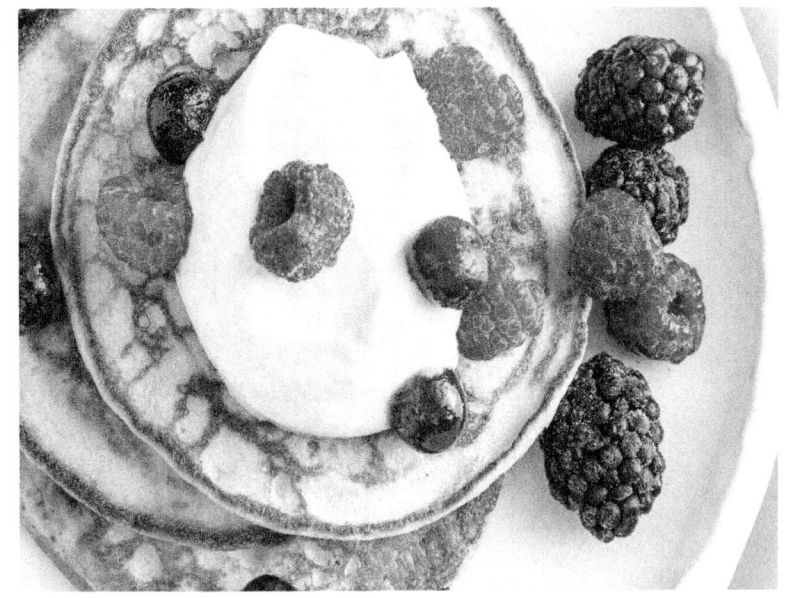

Ingredients

1 Medium Chicken egg

1 tsp Honey

1 scoop of Protein Powder

1 tsp Coconut Oil

1 Banana Mashed

Instructions

1. The pancake is one of the items that may be used in the most diverse ways across the board. I've tried to make this recipe simple by utilizing bananas and whey protein powder flavored with vanilla.
2. If you wish to make this recipe grain-free, omit the muesli and increase the number of nuts and seeds you use in its place. You are also free to exchange/substitute any other sweetener you choose in its place of honey.
3. After blending the banana and egg, you should get a smooth consistency.
4. When adding the protein powder, do it gradually and steadily, smoothing out any lumps that may form along the way.
5. If you want to recreate this stack, you may either use a small frying pan or, for more practical results, pour two to three dollops into a larger skillet. Either way, the stack will be created.
6. On each pancake, spread some honey, sprinkle some muesli, and finish with some sliced banana.

| Nutrition Facts | Calories: 35.5 calories, Proteins: 3.8g, Carbs: 6.5g, Fat: 0.3g |

3.3: Cheddar Zucchini Muffins

Prep Time: 10 minutes

Cook Time: 25 minutes

Servings: 1

Difficulty level: Easy

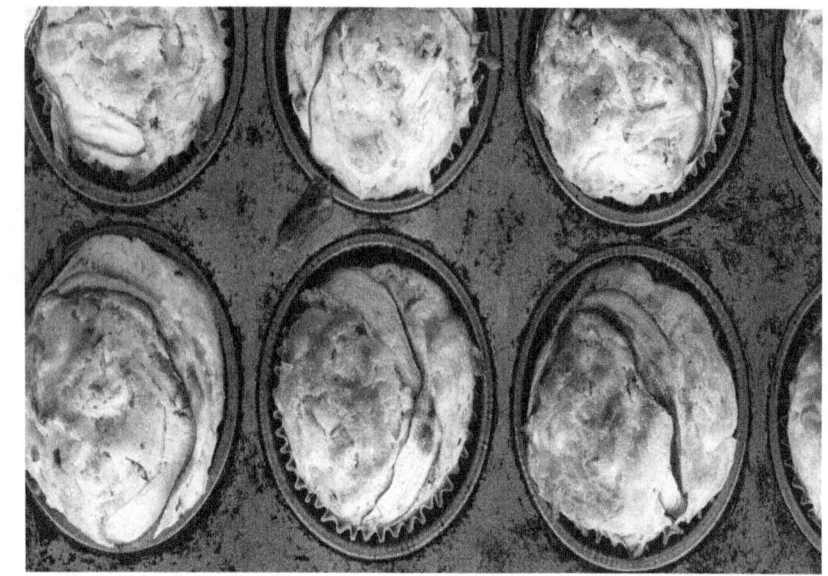

Ingredients

2 tablespoons almond flour	2 ounces zucchini
1/8 tsp baking soda	2 ounces of cheddar cheese
1/8 tsp salt	1/8 tsp black pepper
1/4 tsp garlic powder	1 large egg
1/4 tsp onion powder	

Instructions

1. Raise to a temperature of 350 degrees the temperature in the oven.
2. Flour, egg, baking soda, and spices should all be mixed in a blender. Run the mixture through the blender until it is completely smooth. In addition to the zucchini, include one cup of grated cheese. Pulse the ingredients until the zucchini is evenly dispersed throughout the mixture, but make sure it doesn't become pureed. According to this point of view, the batter should still have distinguishable pieces of green.
3. Place roughly three-quarters of the batter into each cup of a muffin tin that has been lined. On top of it, sprinkle the extra 1 tablespoon of cheese. Bake the muffins for about 25 minutes at 350 degrees Fahrenheit or until a toothpick incorporated into one of the muffins emerges free of any residue.
4. After three to five minutes, remove the muffins from the pot and set them on a wire rack to cool for the remaining time. If the muffins feel lukewarm when touched, they are ready to be separated from the oven. To be consumed when heated.

Nutrition Facts Calories: 196 calories, Proteins: 10g, Carbs: 5g, Fat: 15g

3.4: Hawaiian Hash

Prep Time: 5 minutes

Cook Time: 15 minutes

Servings: 1

Difficulty level: Easy

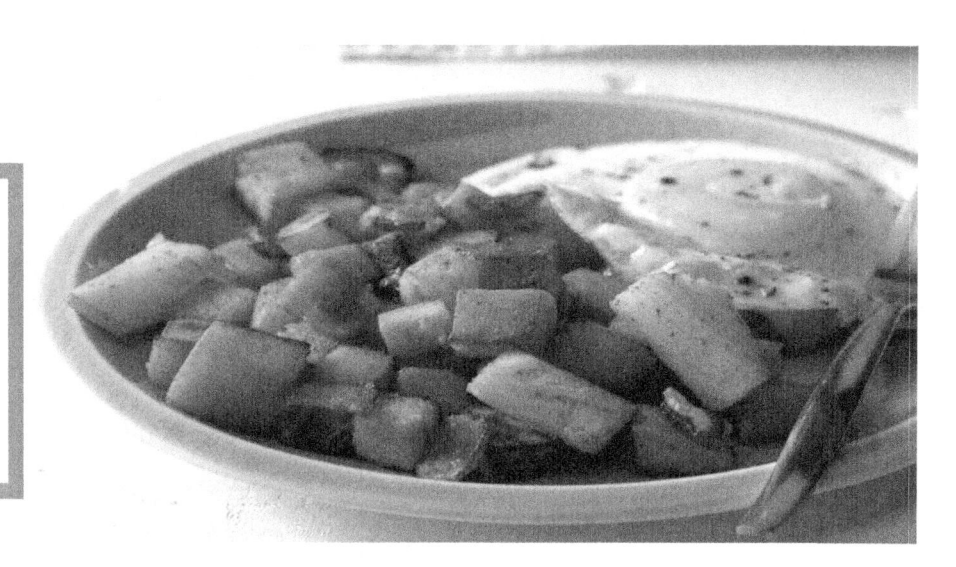

Ingredients

2 tablespoons sweet red pepper	1 tablespoon salsa verde
1 teaspoon cilantro	1/4 cup onion
1/4 cup macadamia nuts	1/4 teaspoon gingerroot
1 cup sweet potatoes	1/4 teaspoon sesame seeds
1/4 teaspoon soy sauce	1 tablespoon water
1/4 cup cubed pineapple	1/4 teaspoon sesame oil
1/4 cup cubed ham	1 teaspoon canola oil

Instructions

1. When heating oils, use a large pan made of cast iron or similar heavy material and heat them over medium-high heat.
2. While the sweet potatoes, onion, pepper, and ginger root cook for five minutes, you should stir them periodically. Add water.
3. Reduce the heat to a low setting, cover the pan, and cook the potatoes for another 8 to 10 minutes while tossing them regularly.
4. After mixing the next five ingredients, cook them while stirring them over medium-high heat for roughly two minutes or until heated.
5. If you choose, top each individual serving with some finely chopped macadamia nuts and chopped cilantro.

Nutrition Facts   Calories: 158 calories, Proteins: 7g, Carbs: 26g, Fat: 4g.

3.5: Mushroom Breakfast Burritos

Prep Time: 10 minutes

Cook Time: 20 minutes

Servings: 1

Difficulty level: Intermediate

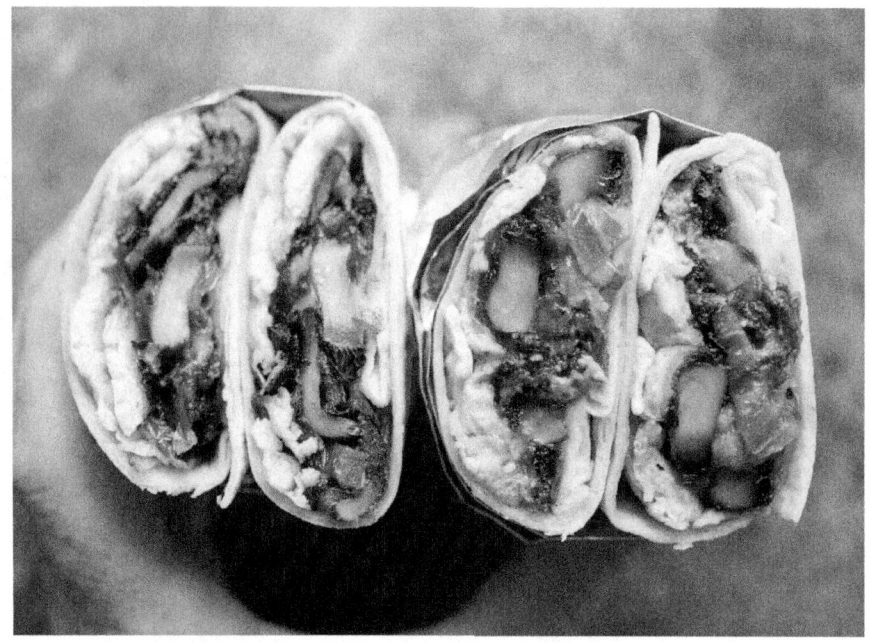

Ingredients

1 cup chopped mushrooms	Salt and pepper
1.5 tablespoons milk	1 tablespoon vegetable oil
1/8 teaspoon salt	2 whole-wheat tortillas
2 cups chopped spinach	Cooking spray
2 tablespoons goat cheese	4 large eggs
1 minced garlic clove	1/4 diced onion

Instructions

1. Oil should be heated over a medium flame.
2. Prepare for two to three minutes.
3. Cook for about 05 minutes or until the mushrooms have become golden brown (about 3-4 minutes).
4. Simply turning the mushrooms over will allow the other side to finish cooking.
5. Put the spinach in the pan and cook it at a simmer for three to four minutes or until it has wilted.
6. Salt the veggies to your liking, then mix them all after seasoning.

7. Take the pan away from where the heat comes from and set it aside.
8. In a large mixing/stirring bowl, merge the flour and the eggs when it comes to flavor, season, to taste.
9. Prepare the third large skillet by heating it over medium heat. Spray the pan with cooking spray, then add the egg mixture.
10. Cook for approximately four to five minutes, stirring the mixture often or until the eggs have reached the desired consistency. Put the burner out of its misery.
11. Warm the tortillas in the microwave for ten seconds to have them ready to use. Spread one and a half tablespoons of goat cheese over the surface of each tortilla that is placed on one of the four pieces of aluminum foil.
12. Distribute the roasted vegetables and scrambled eggs fairly among the four tortillas. After wrapping the bags in foil, put them in the freezer until frozen.
13. When the burritos are ready to eat, remove them from the plastic foil packaging and place them on a plate. In a dish that is safe for the microwave, heat on high for one to two minutes or until the food is well cooked.

Nutrition Facts	Calories: 385 calories, Proteins: 20g, Carbs: 28g, Fat: 22g.

3.6: Cinnamon Apples

Prep Time: 15 minutes

Cook Time: 0 minutes

Servings: 1

Difficulty level: Medium

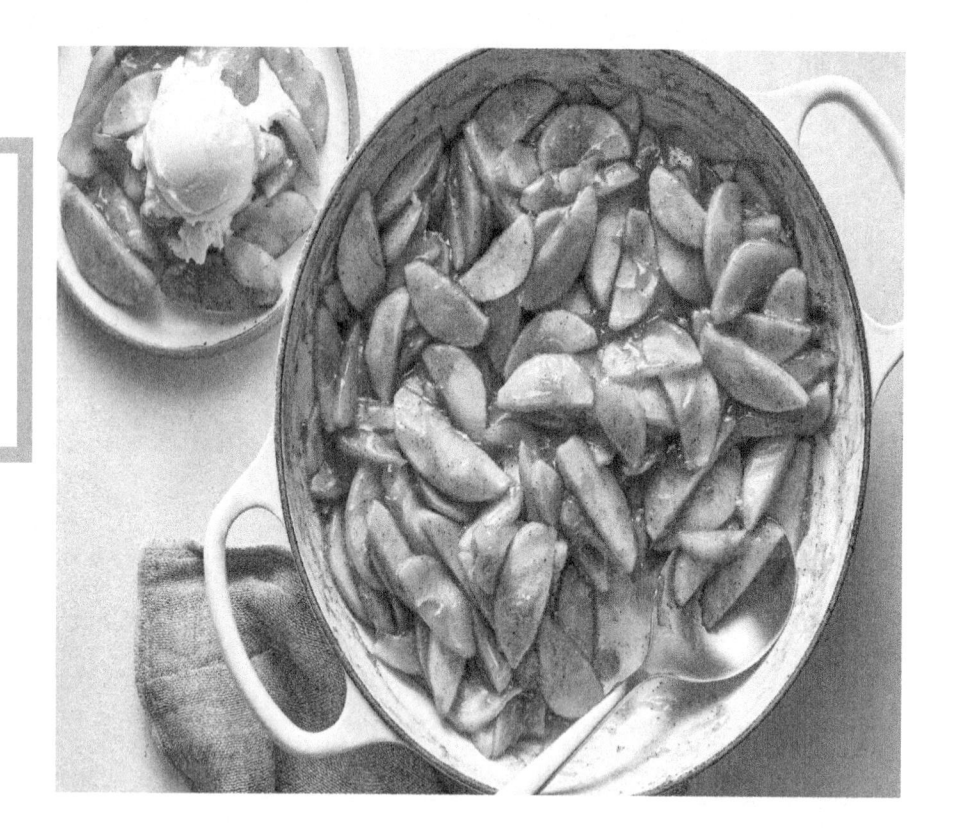

Ingredients

1 heaping tsp maple syrup	3 apples
1 heaping tsp cinnamon	

Instructions

1. Slice, peel, and core the apples.

2. Mix the apples, spices, and maple syrup in the Instant Pot. Add 1/4 cup of water. To immediately coat the apples, stir quickly.

3. 2 minutes of high-pressure cooking. Remove the lid and keep the food warm until ready to serve.

Nutrition Facts   Calories: 130 calories, Proteins: 9g, Carbs: 23g, Fat: 12

3.7: Chia Blueberry Oats

Prep Time: 10 minutes

Cook Time: 15 minutes

Servings: 1

Difficulty level: Medium

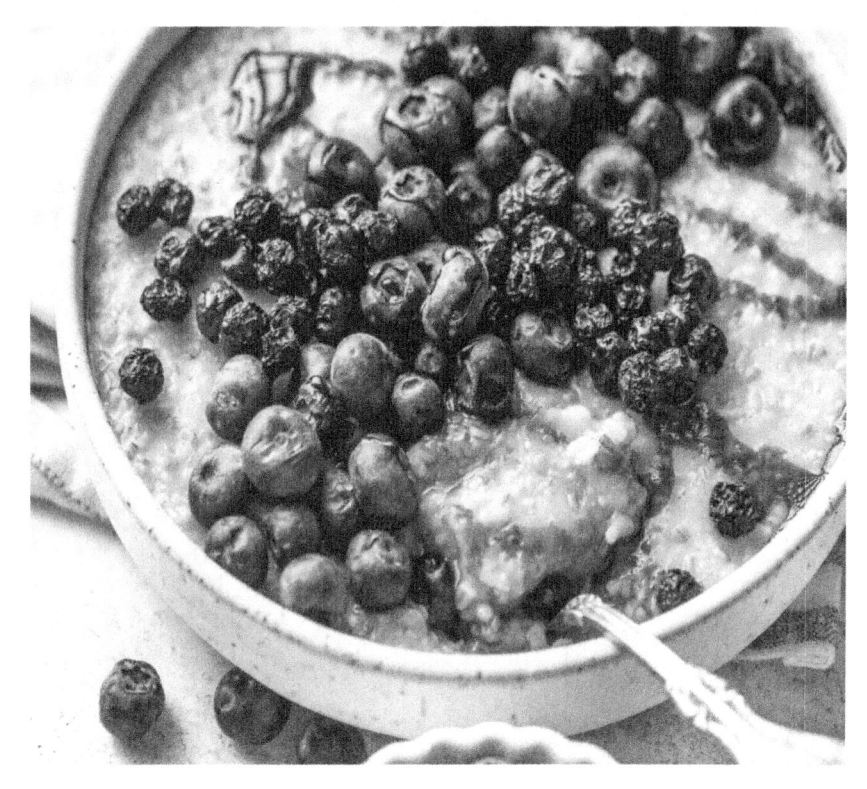

Ingredients

2½ cups unsweetened almond milk	3 tablespoons maple syrup
2 cups rolled oats	2 tablespoons chia seeds
1 cup blueberries	

Instructions

1. Oatmeal, chia seeds, almond milk, and maple syrup should all be combined in a sizable bowl. Mix everything by stirring—place in the refrigerator for the night while wrapped in plastic.

2. Add blueberries the following morning, dividing them into jars and bowls while saving some for topping, if preferred.

3. If preferred, garnish with nuts and coconut flakes before serving and enjoying!

Nutrition Facts   Calories: 150 calories, Proteins: 12g, Carbs: 19g, Fat: 7g

3.7: Avocado Toast with Boiled Eggs

Prep Time: 10 minutes

Cook Time: 15 minutes

Servings: 1

Difficulty level: Medium

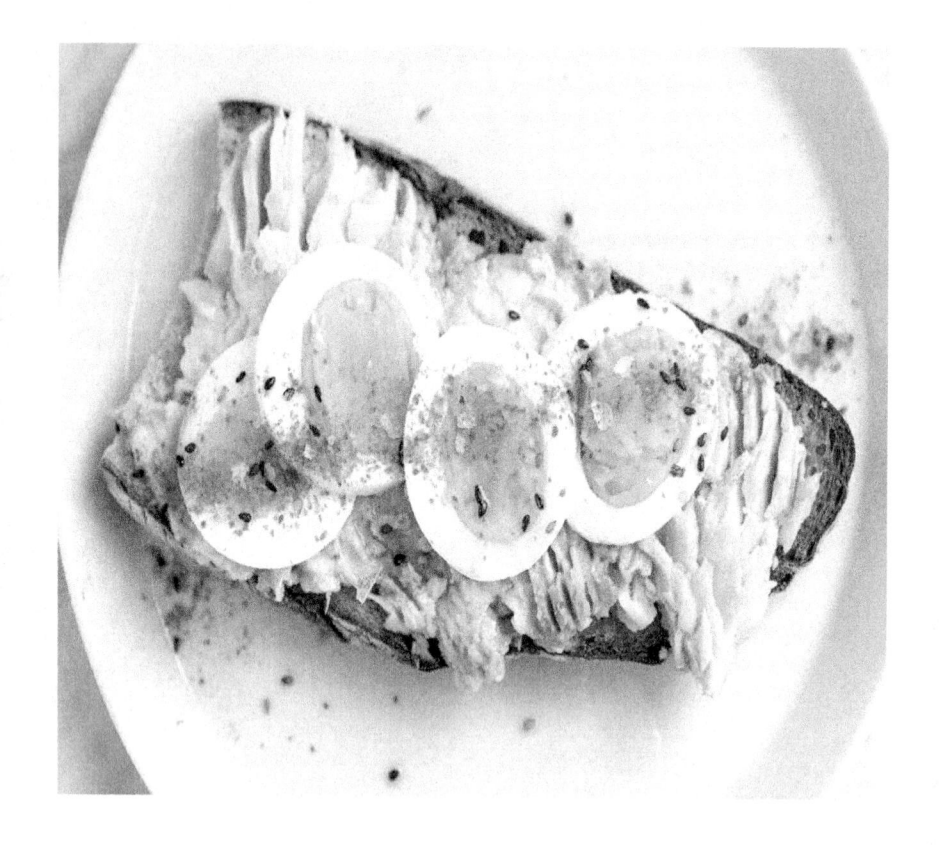

Ingredients

2 avocado

2 boiled eggs

1 whole wheat thin

Instructions

1. In a small saucepan, cover the eggs with water and quickly bring them to a boil. Cook till it desired temperature is reached by reducing the heat to low. After taking them from the water, immediately submerge them in an ice bath to avoid overcooking.

2. Avocados are immediately mashed on the toasted bread.

3. Two tablespoons of chia seeds as a garnish.

Nutrition Facts   Calories: 172 calories, Proteins: 13g, Carbs: 19g, Fat: 10g

3.8: Creamy Oatmeal Porridge

Prep Time: 15 minutes

Cook Time: 15 minutes

Servings: 1

Difficulty level: Medium

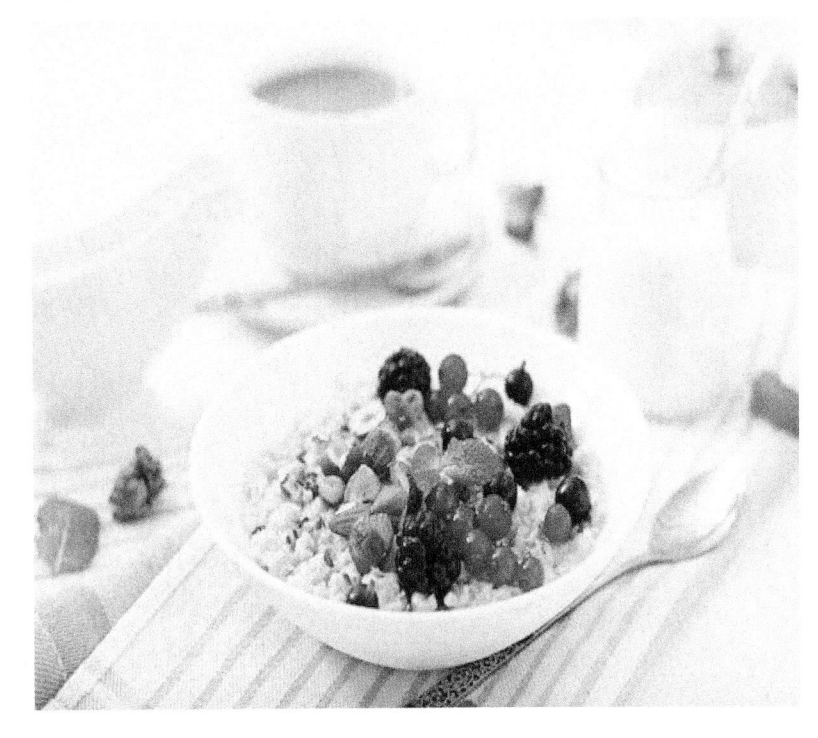

Ingredients

1 cup of oats in rolled form	half a cup of heavy cream
2 ounces of water	1/4 milligram of salt 1/4 cup honey

Instructions

1. The rolled oats, heavy cream, water, and salt should all be combined in a medium-sized pot.

2. Bring mixture to a boil, then decrease the heat and allow it to simmer for about five to seven minutes or until the oats have become soft and creamy.

3. Mix in the honey or whatever sweetener you like.

4. Serve, and have fun with it!

Nutrition Facts   Calories: 348 calories, Proteins: 8g, Carbs: 53g, Fat: 12g

3.9: Blueberry Almond Porridge

Prep Time: 10 minutes Cook

Time: 15 minutes

Servings: 1

Difficulty level: Medium

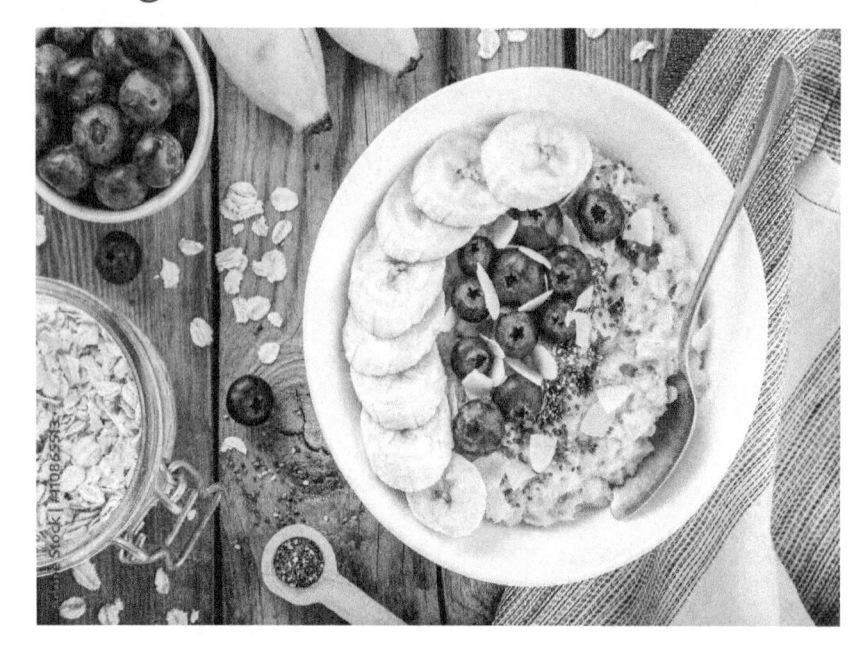

Ingredients

1/2 cup old-fashioned oats	1 cup almond milk
1 tbsp. almond butter	1/2 cup fresh blueberries
1 tsp. vanilla extract	1 tsp. honey
Optional: 1 scoop of protein powder	Pinch of salt

Instructions

1. The almond milk should be heated to boiling in a small saucepan.
2. Mix the oats, salt, and vanilla essence using a stirring motion.
3. Reduce the heat, and cook the oats over a low simmer for about five to seven minutes, stirring the mixture regularly.
4. Honey and almond butter should be stirred together.
5. Fresh blueberries should be sprinkled on top of the cooked oats.
6. Enjoy while it's still hot!

Nutrition Facts   Calories: 372 calories, Proteins: 16g, Carbs: 54g, Fat: 15g

Chapter 4: Snacks and Sides

4.1: Chia Seed Pudding

Prep Time: 60 minutes

Cook Time: 5 minutes

Servings: 1

Difficulty level: Easy

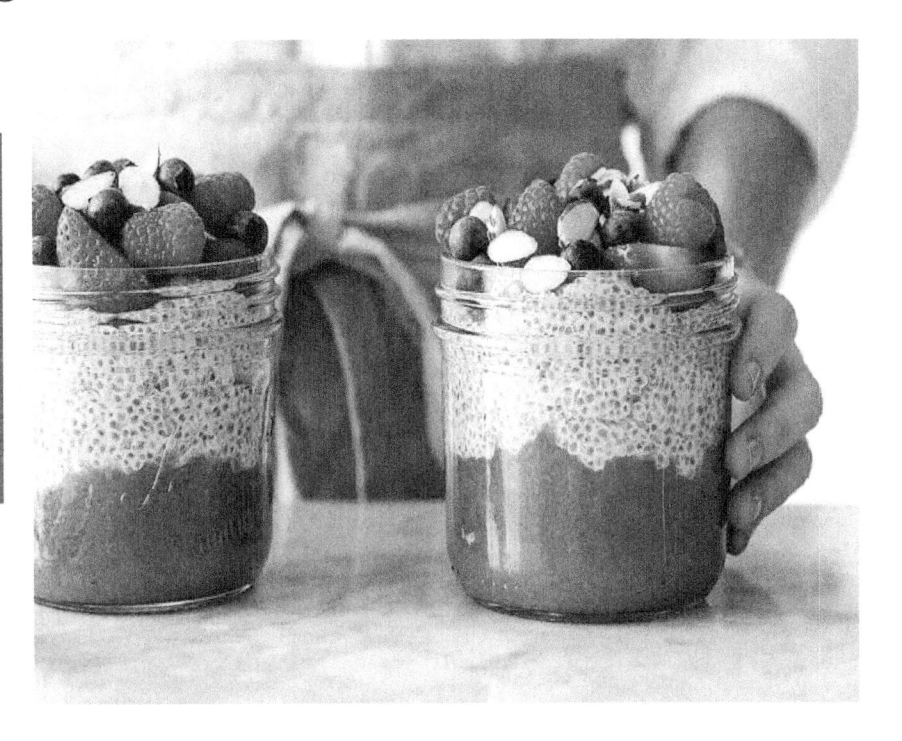

Ingredients

1/4 teaspoon liquid stevia	1/2 teaspoon pumpkin pie spice
3 tablespoons coconut milk	2 tablespoons chia seeds
2 tablespoons pumpkin puree	

Instructions

1. Whisk all items together in a medium mixing basin. Transfer to distinct serving utensils.

2. Put in the cooler for a least two hours to set. Serve chilled and garnish as desired.

Nutrition Facts — Calories: 310 calories, Proteins: 38g, Carbs:12 g, Fat: 3g

4.2: Pumpkin Muffins

Prep Time: 10 minutes

Cook Time: 30 minutes

Servings: 1

Difficulty level: Easy

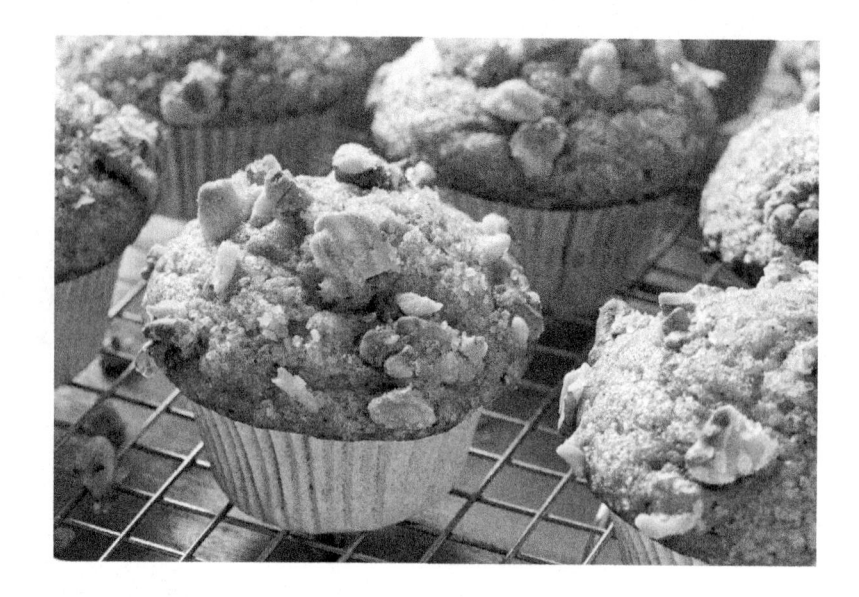

Ingredients

1/12 teaspoon vanilla extract	1/3 tablespoon pure maple syrup
1/6 cup almond flour	1/12 teaspoon baking soda
1 egg	2 tablespoons pumpkin puree
1/12 teaspoon cinnamon	2 tablespoons chocolate chips
1/24 teaspoon nutmeg	1/24 teaspoon sea salt
2 tablespoons Greek yogurt	

Instructions

1. Set a muffin tray aside, oil it, and preheat the oven to 375°F.
2. In a small bowl, add the wet ingredients and stir to blend thoroughly.
3. In a large container, mix the dehydrated ingredients first, then add the liquid ones. After thoroughly combining, add the chocolate chunks.
4. Fill buttered muffin cups with the mixture, and bake for 18 to 22 minutes or until the toothpick comes out clean.
5. It is advised to bake small muffins for 18 minutes so they will cook more quickly. Please keep it in the refrigerator in an airtight container for up to a week. They may be frozen; thaw in the oven for 30 seconds before eating.

Nutrition Facts   Calories: 49 calories, Proteins: 1.7g, Carbs: 6.6 g, Fat: 2g

4.3: Keto Soft Pretzels

Prep Time: 25 minutes

Cook Time: 10 minutes

Servings: 1

Difficulty level: Easy

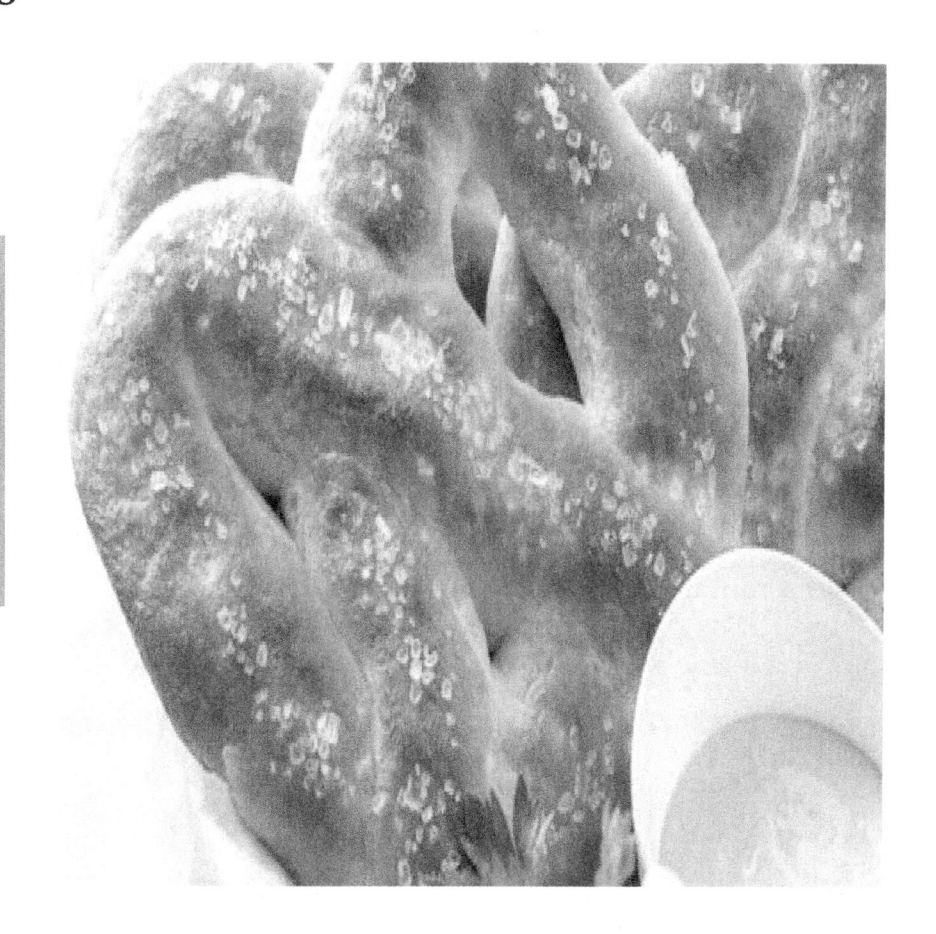

Ingredients

1/2 oz cream cheese

1 teaspoon melted butter

1/12 teaspoon psyllium husk powder

1 large egg beaten

1 tablespoon warm water

1/12 teaspoon yeast

2 tablespoons almond flour

1/24 teaspoon coarse kosher salt

1/12 teaspoon baking powder

1/8 cup mozzarella cheese

Instructions

1. Prepare a large roasting tray by coating it with parchment or a Silpat liner and preheating the oven to 425 degrees Fahrenheit.

2. Mix the yeast and the warm water in a small dish by stirring them with a fork; then, set the bowl aside for five to ten minutes.

3. In the meanwhile, in a separate bowl, combine the ground almonds, psyllium fiber powder, and baking powder. Set this mixture aside.

4. Combine the mozzarella with cream cheese and melt it in the microwave or a double boiler. If you are melting the cheese in the microwave, start heating it for one minute, mix it with a fork, and continue cooking it in 15-second increments until it is completely melted.

5. First, incorporate the yeast that has been dissolved into the cheese mixture. Next, stir in the egg, and lastly, stir in the combination of almond flour and salt. It is easiest to accomplish this using your hands; to prevent the bread from sticking to your hands while you knead the ingredients together after they form a dough, gently spritz your hands with some avocado or olive oil and then knead the ingredients together.

6. Cut each piece of dough into four equal parts, roll each piece into a log that is about 4 inches long, and then cut each log into four bite-sized pieces.

7. Arrange the bits in a single layer on the baking sheet that has been prepared, and bake for about ten minutes or until brown.

8. As quickly as they emerge from the oven, delicately brush some melted butter on top of each pretzel, nibble and then sprinkle some salt.

9. Before serving, let the dish gently cool.

| **Nutrition Facts** | Calories: 171 calories, Proteins: 9g, Carbs: 4g, Fat: 13g |

4.4: Spinach Artichoke Dip

Prep Time: 10 minutes

Cook Time: 45 minutes

Servings: 1

Difficulty level: Easy

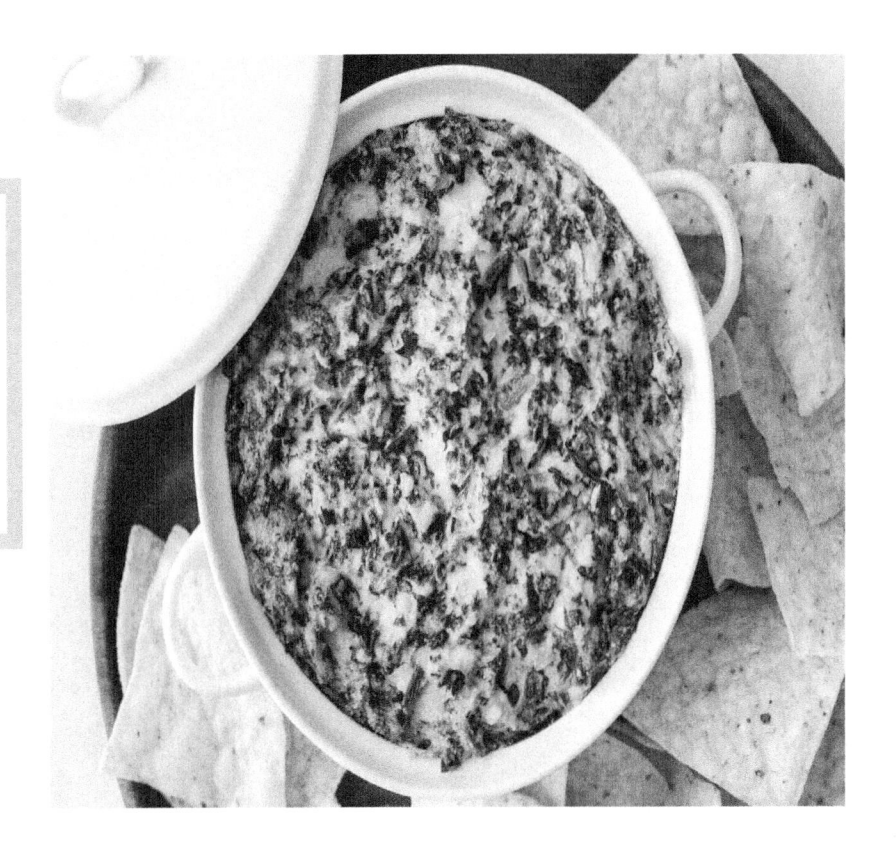

Ingredients

2 tablespoons shredded fontina cheese

2 tablespoons grated parmesan cheese

8 ounces spinach

1/4 can artichoke hearts

2 tablespoons plain yogurt

1 clove garlic

1/72 teaspoon black pepper

2 tablespoons avocado mayo

1/72 teaspoon salt

Instructions

1. Turn the oven on to 350 degrees.

2. After it has been defrosted, frozen spinach should be squeezed to remove any extra moisture. When I thaw food in the microwave, I often use a big glass dish to contain the food. Afterward, squeeze the water out of the spinach using either a towel or a dish towel. Because it contains a lot of liquid, you want to make it as dry as possible. When you are finished, it seems like a massive clump!

3. Empty the water from the artichoke can before using it. The artichoke sections should all be cut in half lengthwise.

4. Combine the mayonnaise, yogurt, salt, garlic, and parmesan cheese in a stick or high-powered blender. Add one-third of the artichoke hearts to the mixture. Mix until everything is evenly distributed.

5. After that, add the rest of the artichoke hearts, followed by the spinach, and finish with the fontina cheese.

6. I used a dish that was 1.5 quarts/1.5 liters in capacity and spread the mixture evenly before placing it in the oven.

7. Add a quarter cup's worth of shredded feta cheese on top.

8. Bake in a heated oven for 20 minutes while covered with aluminum foil, then remove the foil and bake for 20-25 minutes.

9. To gently brown the top of the dip, place it under the broiler for about five minutes after the oven has been set to broil. Be careful since the broiler works quite quickly. It might take you anything from one to five minutes to finish yours!

Nutrition Facts   Calories: 139 calories, Proteins: 2g, Carbs:6 g, Fat:11g

4.5: Chocolate Peanut Butter Bites

Prep Time: 30 minutes

Cook Time: 10 minutes

Servings: 1

Difficulty level: Easy

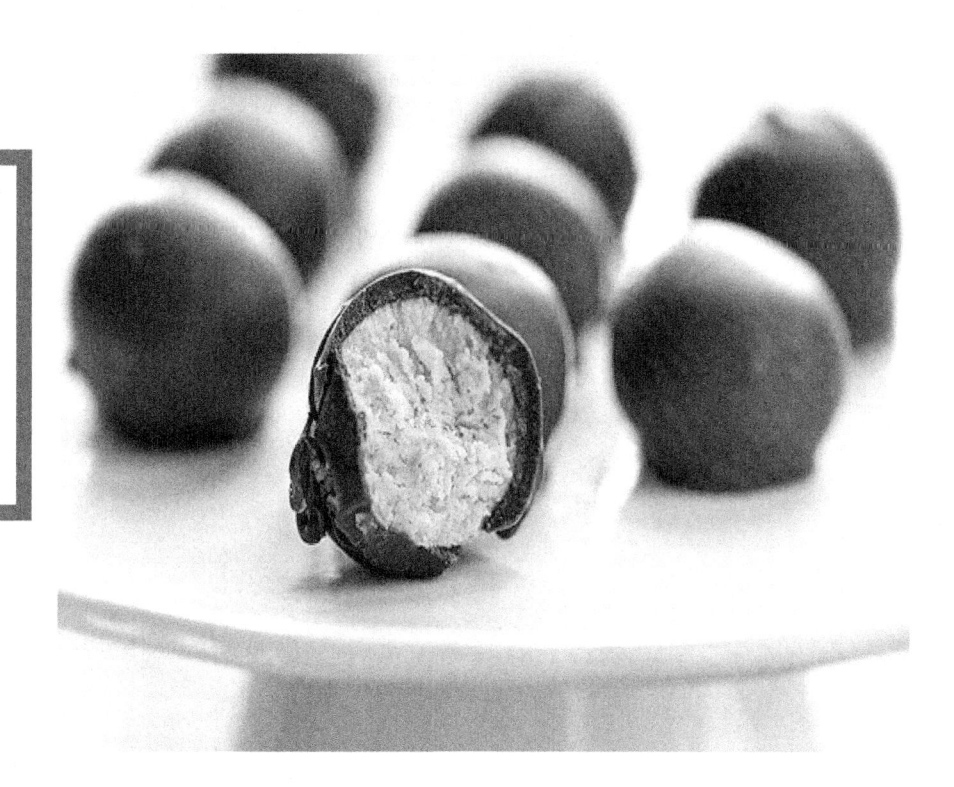

Ingredients

2 tablespoons dark chocolate chips	2 tablespoons peanut butter
2 tablespoons pitted dates	1 teaspoon cacao powder
1/8 can of black beans	1 scoop of chocolate protein powder
1/4 teaspoon sea salt	

Instructions

1. It is important to line a baking sheet with parchment paper before beginning.

2. Put the dates, black beans, cocoa protein powder, nut kinds of butter, kosher salt, and cacao powder into the food processor bowl and pulse until everything is combined. The mixture should be processed in the food processor until perfectly smooth, with occasional stops to scrape the sides.

3. To bake the cookies, form the dough into balls with a diameter of about one inch and residence

them on a lubricated baking sheet. It should result in around 20 balls.

4. The chocolate drizzle may be made by melting white chocolate in a dual boiler and then sprinkling it over the balls when cooled. This step is completely voluntary.

5. Please put them in the freezer for at least an hour, or put them inside the refrigerator for about an hour so that they may become firm. Enjoy!

Nutrition Facts	Calories: 212 calories, Proteins: 2g, Carbs:6 g, Fat:13

4.6: Cinnamon Apple Porridge

Prep Time: 10 minutes

Cook Time: 10 minutes

Servings: 1

Difficulty level: Easy

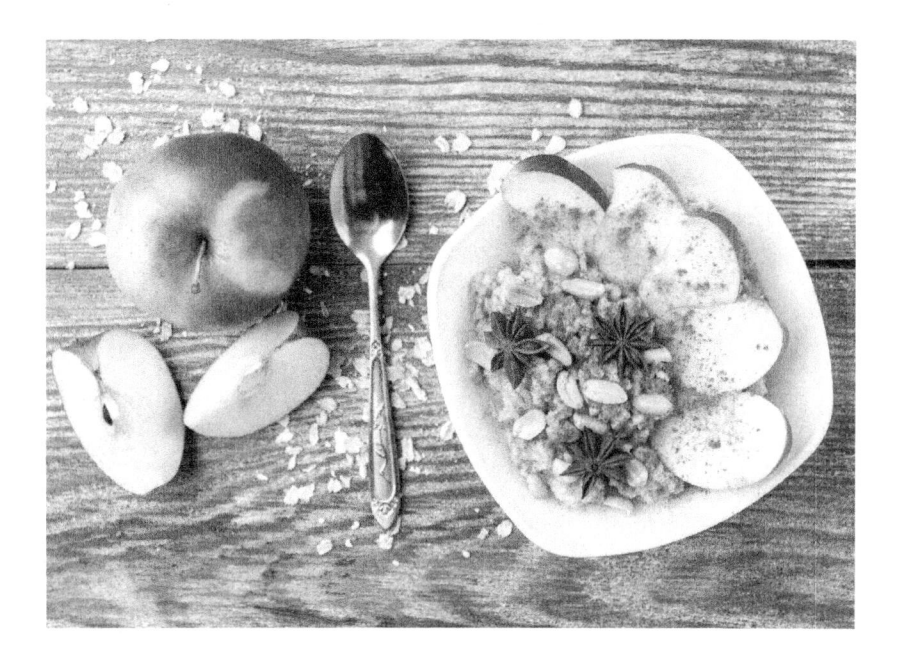

Ingredients

1/2 cup old-fashioned oats	1 cup water
1 medium apple, diced	1 tsp. cinnamon
1 tbsp. maple syrup	1 tsp. vanilla extract
Pinch of salt	Optional: 1 scoop of protein powder

Instructions

1. Bring tap water to a boil in a saucepan of a manageable size.

2. Mix the oats, salt, and vanilla essence using a stirring motion.

3. Reduce the heat, and cook the oats over a low simmer for about five to seven minutes, stirring the mixture regularly.

4. Mix in the chopped apple, cinnamon, and maple syrup until everything is well combined.

5. Enjoy while it's still hot!

Nutrition Facts   Calories: 267 calories, Proteins: 6g, Carbs: 59g, Fat: 3g

4.7: Tuna Salad Stuffed Tomatoes

Prep Time: 12 minutes

Cook Time: 15 minutes

Servings: 1

Difficulty level: Medium

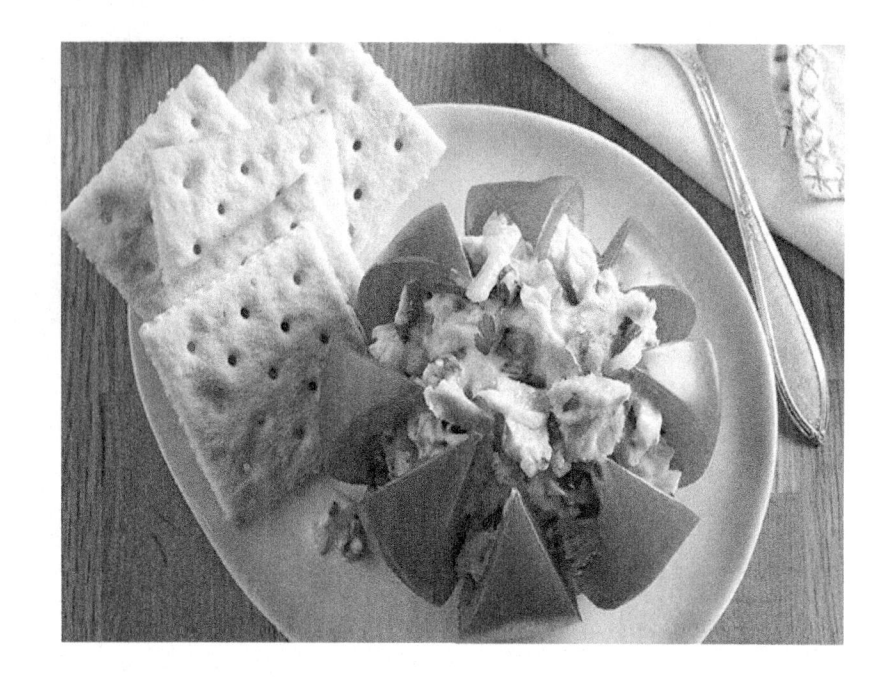

Ingredients

2 cans of chunk light tuna in water, drained	1/4 cup mayonnaise
1/4 cup plain Greek yogurt	1 tsp. Dijon mustard
Salt and pepper, to taste	4 large tomatoes
1/4 cup chopped fresh basil	

Instructions

1. In a large bowl, combine the tuna that has been drained together with the mayonnaise, Greek yogurt, Dijon mustard, and the seasonings of your choice.

2. Remove the tomato tops and use a spoon to scoop out the seeds and meat from the tomatoes.

3. When the tomatoes have been hollowed out, fill them with tuna salad.

4. The filled tomatoes would benefit from having some chopped basil sprinkled on top.

5. Enjoy the filled tomatoes best when they are served chilly.

Nutrition Facts   Calories: 360 calories, Proteins: 35g, Carbs: 12g, Fat: 20g

4.8: Turkey, Avocado, and Cheddar Wrap

Prep Time: 20 minutes

Cook Time: 20 minutes

Servings: 1

Difficulty level: Medium

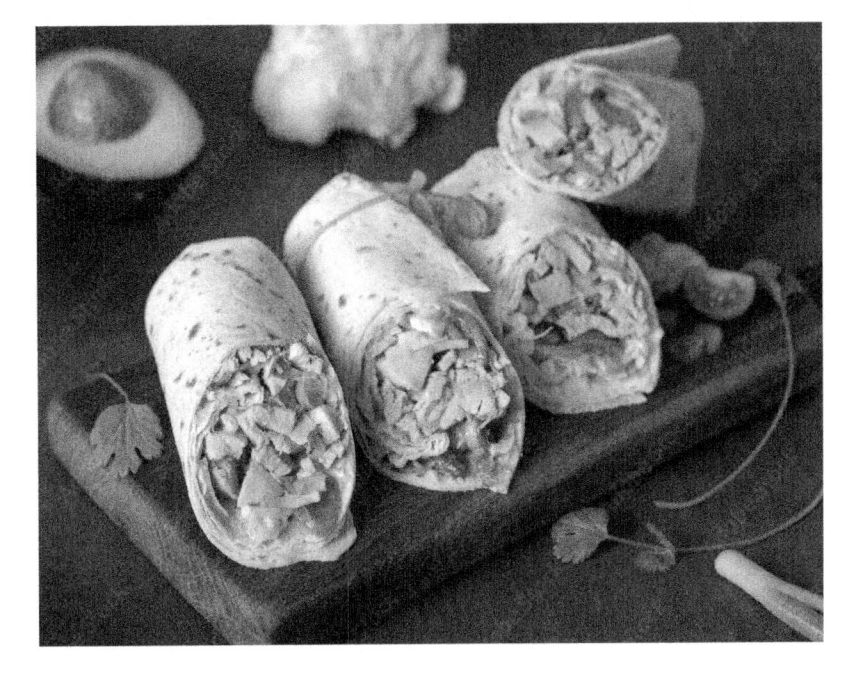

Ingredients

4 whole wheat tortillas	4 oz. thinly sliced turkey breast
1/2 cup shredded cheddar cheese	2 ripe avocados, pitted and mashed
4 lettuce leaves	Salt and pepper, to taste

Instructions

1. In a microwave-safe bowl, cook the tortillas made from whole wheat for about 15 to 20 seconds or until they are warm and flexible.
2. Spread an equal quantity of mashed avocado on each tortilla, then layer each with sliced turkey breast.
3. The turkey should be covered with shredded cheddar cheese before serving.
4. On top of the cheese, a leaf of lettuce should be placed.
5. Salt and pepper may be added to taste as a seasoning.
6. To make a wrap out of the tortilla, roll it up firmly and tuck it in the ends.
7. You may serve the wrap right once or wrap it in plastic and store it in the refrigerator for later.

Nutrition Facts   Calories: 478 calories, Proteins: 30g, Carbs: 38g, Fat: 27g

4.9: Shrimp Kabobs

Prep Time: 10 minutes

Cook Time: 15 minutes

Servings: 1

Difficulty level: Medium

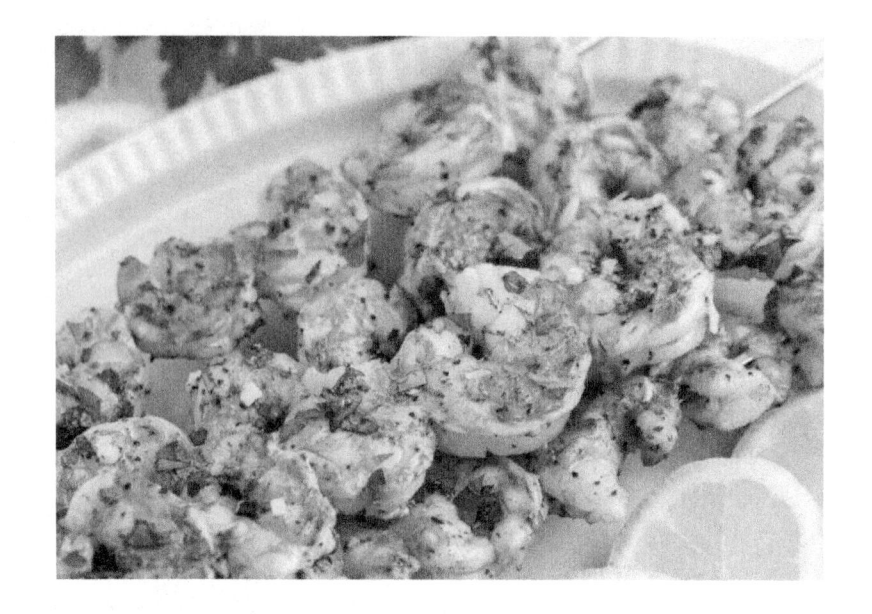

Ingredients

1.33 lbs shrimp	1/4 cup freshly squeezed lemon juice
4 cloves garlic	2 tbsp butter
2 tbsp parsley	Salt and pepper

Instructions

1. Either preheat the grill or the stove to 450 degrees.

2. Butter should be added to a small pan. Add the garlic, lime juice, and Italian spice after it has melted. Cook the garlic on low for 2 to 3 minutes until fragrant.

1. Shrimp are threaded onto skewers. Add salt and pepper to taste. Place on a sheet pan and in the oven for 5 to 6 minutes or until pink and well done. Place immediately on the grill to cook on each side for 2-3 seconds until opaque and well cooked.

2. Brush the cooked shrimp with the garlicky butter mixture before serving.

Nutrition Facts	Calories: 134 calories, Proteins: 34g, Carbs: 34g, Fat: 3g

4.10: Grilled Chicken with Vegetables

Prep Time: 15 minutes

Cook Time: 10 minutes

Servings: 1

Difficulty level: Easy

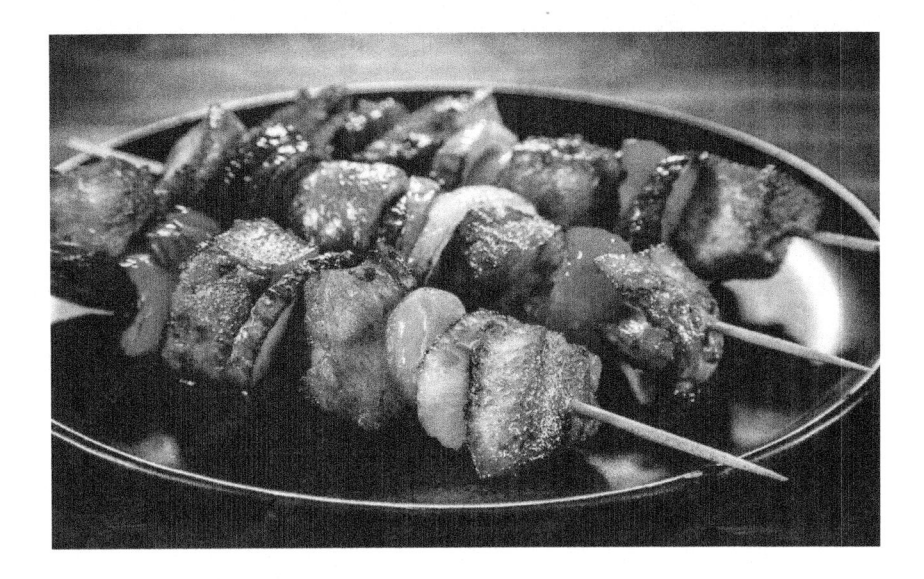

Ingredients

4 boneless, skinless chicken breasts	1 tbsp. olive oil
1 large zucchini, sliced	Salt and pepper, to taste
1 large yellow squash, sliced	1 red bell pepper, sliced
1 large onion, sliced	1 tbsp. dried thyme

Instructions

1. Prepare the grill by heating it to a medium-high temperature.
2. Olive oil, salt, and pepper are the seasonings that should be used on chicken breasts.
3. Place the chicken on the grill & cook for six to eight minutes on each side or until the chicken is cooked through completely.
4. Toss the sliced zucchini, yellow squash, red bell pepper, and onion in a large bowl prepared with dried thyme.
5. Put the veggies on the grill and cook them for about five to seven minutes or until they are soft and have a little char.
6. Chicken and veggies that have been grilled should be served together.

Nutrition Facts Calories: 385 calories, Proteins: 43g, Carbs: 13g, Fat: 17g

Invite to Review Book

I am grateful that you took the time to read my book. I hope that you found it to be both pleasant and educational. As an author, I place a high value on the comments and suggestions made by my readers, and I would be very interested in hearing your opinions regarding the book.

If you get a chance, I'd appreciate it if you could leave a review on the platform of your choice whenever you get a chance. Your review has the potential to assist other readers in locating the book in question and making an educated choice regarding whether or not to read it.

I very much appreciate any comments, recommendations, or criticisms that you may have, and I will do my best to incorporate them into future revisions. I am grateful you took the time to read my book, and I look forward to hearing from you soon.

With warmest regards,

Angela Ramsey

Chapter 5: Lunch Recipes

5.1: High-Protein Chicken Soup

Prep Time: 10 minutes

Cook Time: 10 minutes

Servings: 1

Difficulty level: Easy

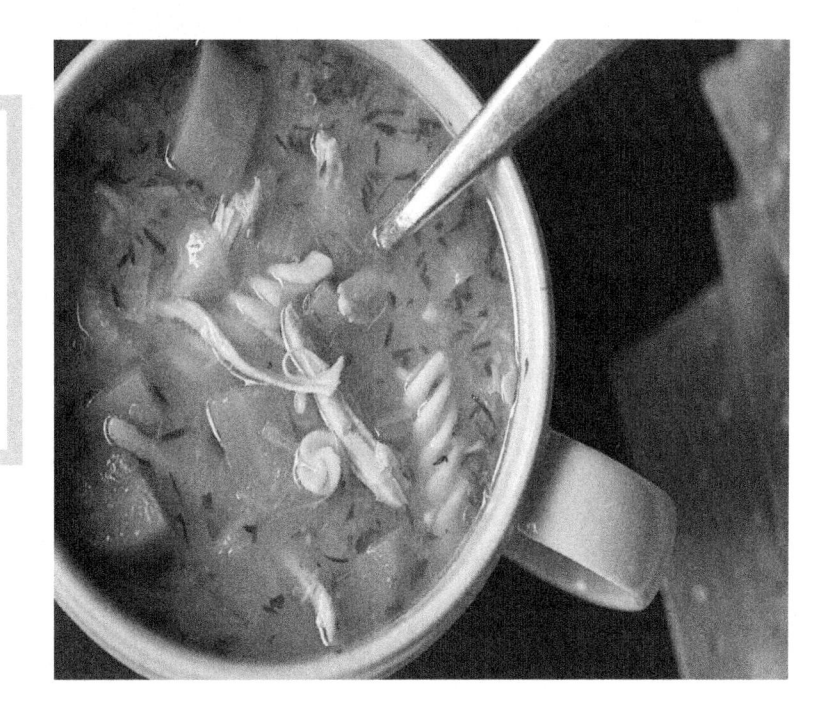

Ingredients

| 4-8 ounces of bone broth | Protein Meal Replacement |

Instructions

1. Place anything from four to eight liters of chicken soup in the shaker cup.

2. Heat for approximately forty seconds in the microwaves (or until the water reaches 140 degrees Fahrenheit or less; protein will begin to lump at temperatures over 140 degrees Fahrenheit).

3. After adding the chicken soup protein powder and giving it a shake, you may enjoy it.

4. Be careful when opening the lid of the shaker cup due to pressure from heat because it may cause a mess.

Nutrition Facts Calories: 210 calories, Proteins: 37g, Carbs:11 g, Fat:2g

5.2: Baked Ricotta

Prep Time: 5 minutes

Cook Time: 30 minutes

Servings: 1

Difficulty level: Easy

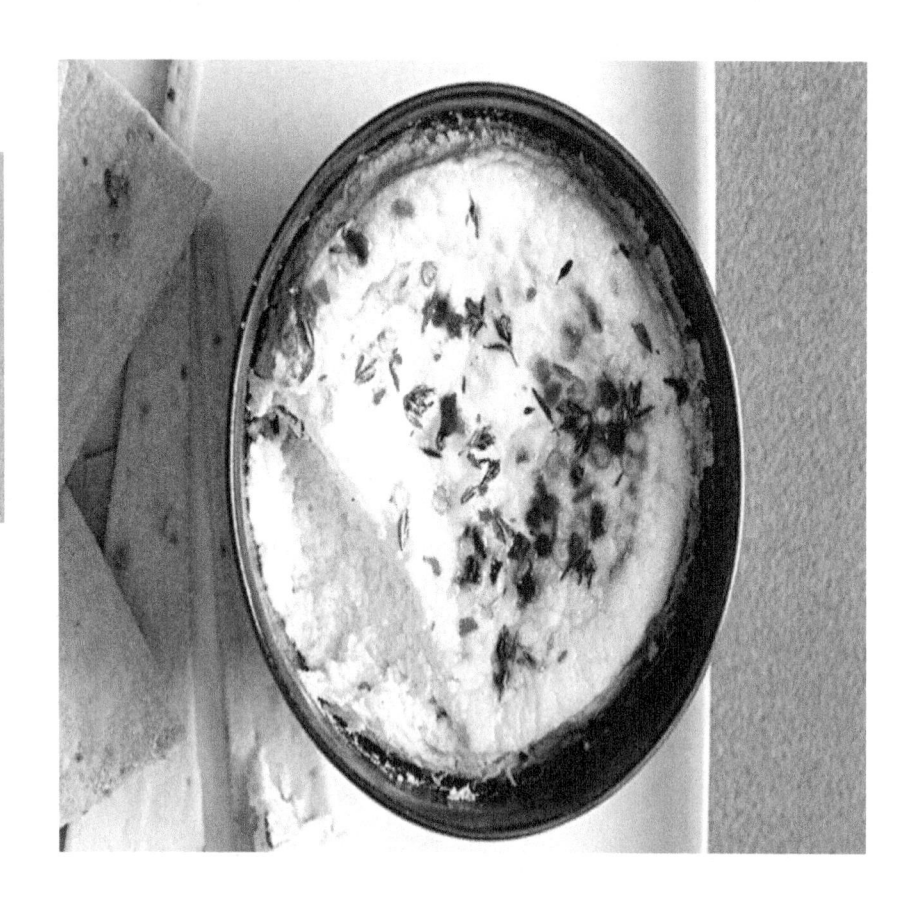

Ingredients

1/2 cup + 1/2 tablespoon parmesan cheese grated	1 large egg
1/48 teaspoon red pepper flakes	8 oz whole milk ricotta cheese
1 tablespoon chives thinly sliced	

Instructions

1. Prepare the oven by preheating it to 400 degrees. To coat the baking dish, use butter or a spray that prevents sticking.

2. Ricotta, eggs, one cup of grated parmesan, two tablespoons of chopped chives, and one-fourth of a teaspoon of crushed red pepper should be mixed in a various containers basin. Use a spatula to stir the ingredients until they are completely incorporated.

3. Ricotta and parmesan cheeses combined and placed in a bowl.

4. Place the ricotta mixture in the dish prepared for baking (es).

5. On top, sprinkle the rest of the grated parmesan cheese, then put the dish into the oven to bake for about half an hour or until the Ricotta has become golden brown and risen to the top like a soufflé.

6. Ricotta in little cocottes, before being baked, can be served with spoons or as an accompaniment to crudités, crostini, salami, or fresh fruit.

7. Notes Start checking the baked Ricotta at the 15-minute mark if you want a cheese dip that is less cooked than average.

8. It won't be golden brown or bubbled out, it will nevertheless be safe to eat (the eggs will be cooked all the way through), and you may serve it with bruschetta, crudité, fruit, or whatever else you choose.

9. In its unbaked form, Ricotta can be stored in the refrigerator for over three months, after which it can be baked under the directions given above, with a few extra minutes added.

Nutrition Facts	Calories: 310 calories, Proteins: 38g, Carbs:12 g, Fat: 3g

5.3: Butterfly Chicken

Prep Time: 10 minutes

Cook Time: 10 minutes

Servings: 1

Difficulty level: Easy

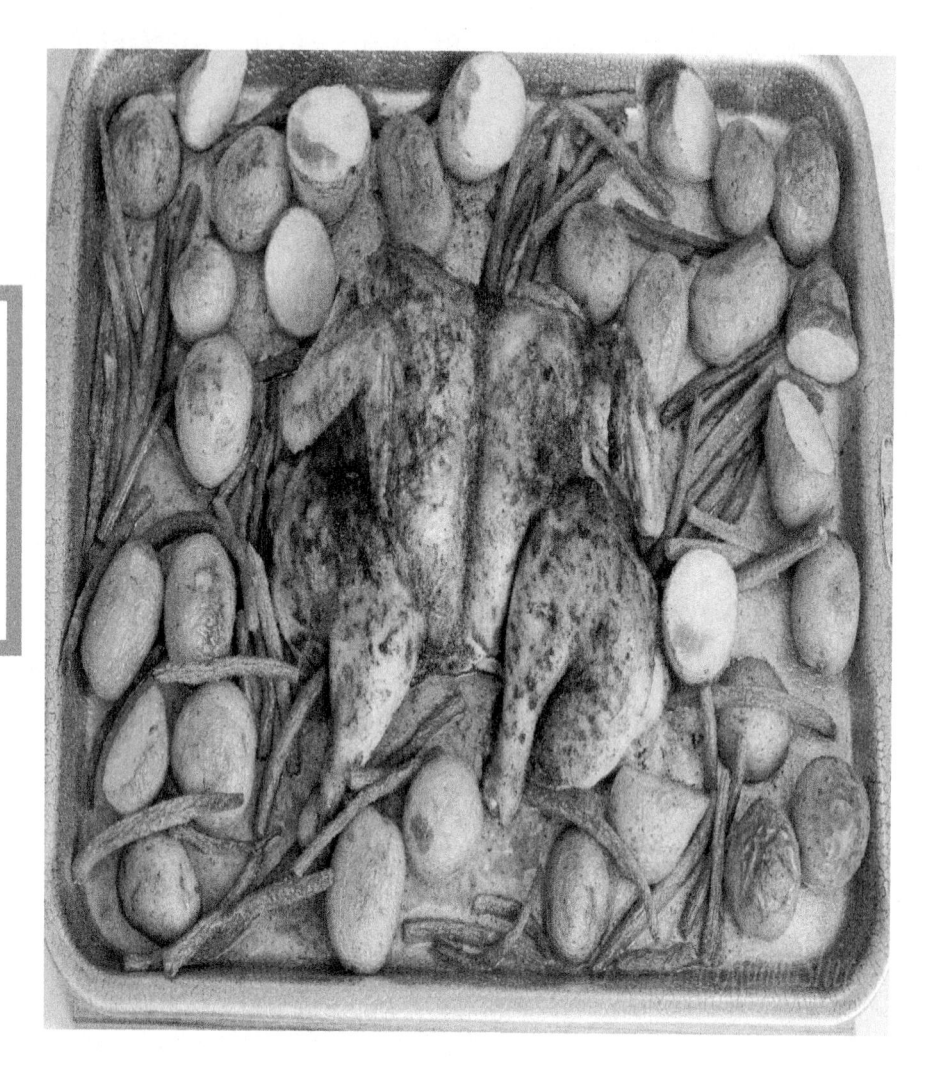

Ingredients

2 large eggs	2 tablespoon cilantro
Pepper	6 boneless chicken breasts
1 tablespoon turmeric	Salt
3 garlic cloves, minced	

Instructions

1. First, make four shallow slashes across the top of every chicken breast. Next, season both sides of the chicken breasts with salt and pepper. Because of this, the marinade taste will infiltrate the meat more quickly, and the chicken breasts will be able to cook more quickly and evenly.

2. After that, combine fresh lime juice, garlic that has been minced, and cilantro that has been chopped in a big bowl, and then add the chicken breasts to the marinade. Cover the mixing bowl and let it sit at room temperature for approximately thirty minutes.

3. Use a fork to give the eggs a good beating in a bowl. Mix the turmeric powder and panko or wheat crumbs in a separate bowl.

4. Place every chicken breast in the bowl containing the beaten eggs, and turn them into an egg. After that, use the mixture of bread crumbs and turmeric to cover both sides of every chicken breast.

5. Cook the chicken breasts over medium heat in a large nonstick skillet for approximately 6–10 minutes on each side, using half the amount the vegetable oil called for in the recipe. To prevent the breadcrumbs from burning, wipe the skillet well with a clean towel between each batch, if necessary. Preparing food in several stages is essential to prevent the pan from becoming too crowded, which would cause the temperature to drop.

6. After the chicken has been cooked through (there should be no hint of pink), transfer it to a big platter lined with two layers of paper towel to soak up a little of the oil. You can serve it in a sandwich, topped with the raw mango salsa, alongside roasted or boiled vegetables of your choosing, or you can roast or steam them yourself.

7. Remember that any leftovers must be stowed in the freezer and covered for up to two days.

Nutrition Facts	Calories: 230 calories, Proteins: 25g, Carbs:18 g, Fat:6g

5.4: Vegetable Khichdi

Prep Time: 10 minutes

Cook Time: 15 minutes

Servings: 1

Difficulty level: Easy

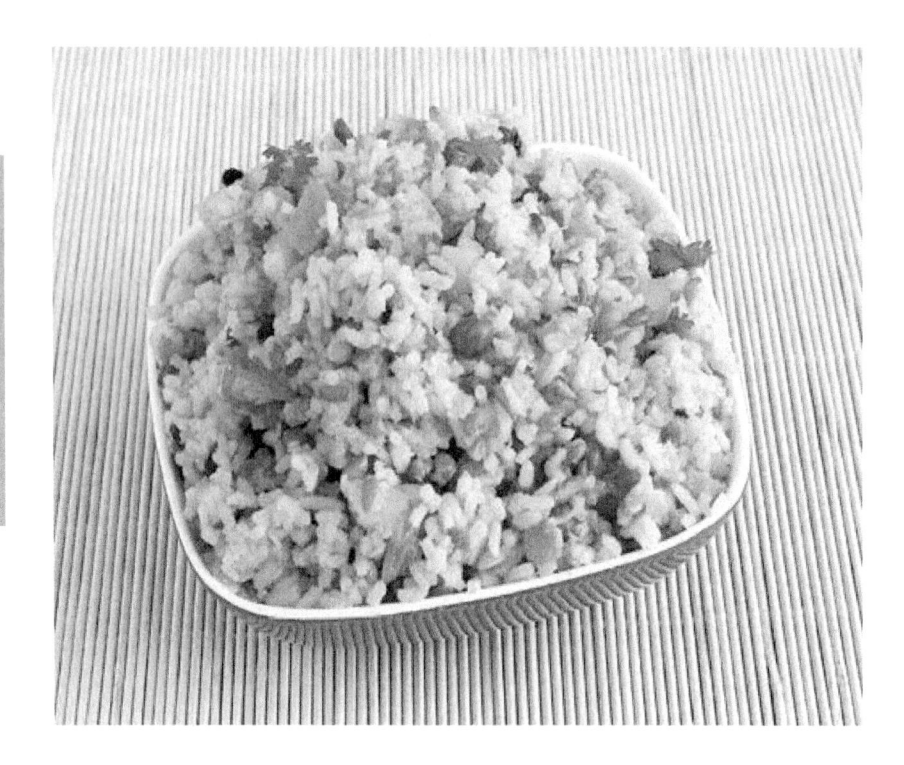

Ingredients

1/2 medium onion chopped	1 1/2 teaspoons ghee
1/2 teaspoon ginger	1 green chili
1 1/2 cups water	1/2 cup chopped spinach
1/4 cup white rice (short grain)	

Instructions

1. When using the Instant Pot, select the SAUTE mode. Put some ghee or oil in the Crock Pot. Note: Ghee enhances the flavor of the dish.

2. After the saucepan has reached a high temperature, put in the cumin (tax is a levy), garlic, and green chilies, and saute for a minute and a half.

3. Cumin and chiles will be sauteed in the next step. Collage

4. Mix in the finely chopped onion. Sauté the onions until their color changes to a light brown.

5. Step to sauté onions till they have broken down completely.

6. Then, after a minute of cooking, add the mixed veggies and the spinach.

7. Step to add spinach and other veggies to the collage.

8. After that, put in the rice, the rinsed dal, the red chili powder, the turmeric powder, the coriander powder, and the water. Combine thoroughly.

9. The next step is to add the rice, moong dal, and water collage. Turn the pressure regulator to the Sealing position, then close the Instant Pot. Prepare using High Pressure for a total of 8 minutes. When the timer on the pot goes off, wait for the tension to release naturally (NPR).

10. Step to pressure college cook for a total of 8 minutes.

11. After the pressure has been released, the lid should be opened, the cilantro should be added, and the khichdi should be thoroughly mixed.

12. Note: If the rice is still firm but not mushy, select the saute mode, pour in a half teaspoon of water, and continue cooking for one more minute.

13. Step to add more water, then bring the collage to a boil.

14. Vegetable Solid or liquid form recipe or Mix Vegetable Lentil The rice is finished cooking; it goes well with yogurt, raita, or kadhi.

| **Nutrition Facts** | Calories:350 calories, Proteins: 23g, Carbs:13 g, Fat:4g |

5.5: Tuna Sandwich

Prep Time: 20 minutes

Cook Time: 5 minutes

Servings: 1

Difficulty level: Easy

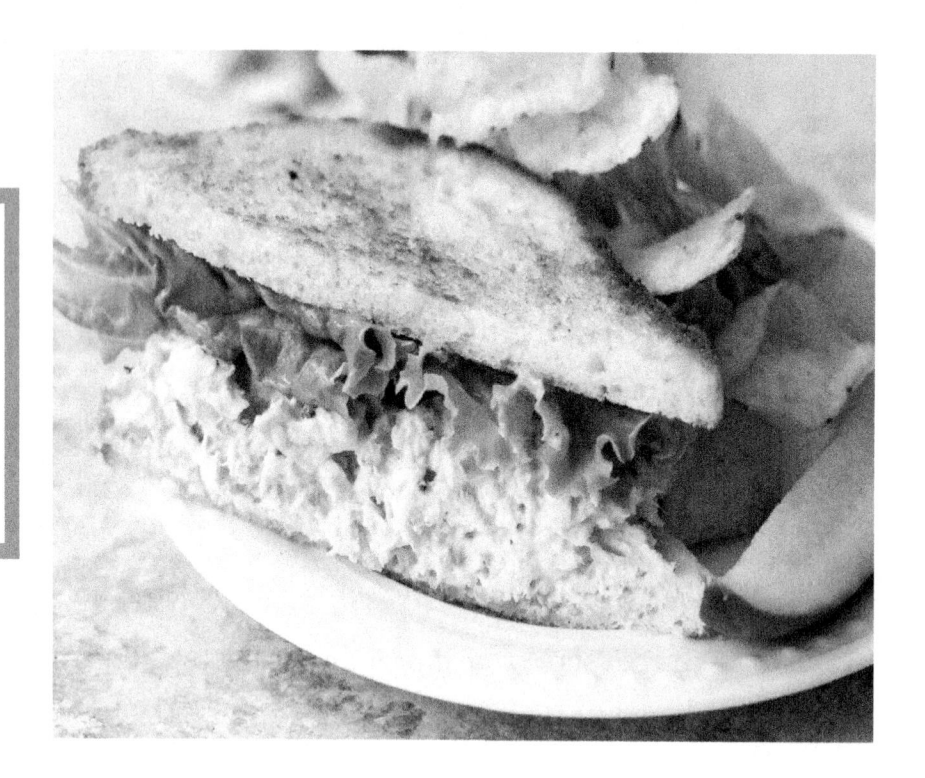

Ingredients

1 apple	8 slices whole-grain bread
1 can 12-oz chunk light tuna	2 tablespoons yogurt
2 tablespoons mayonnaise	1/2 cup raisins
1/4 cup walnuts	1/8 teaspoon ground black pepper
2 tablespoons fresh parsley	1/2 teaspoon curry powder
8 leaves lettuce	

Instructions

1. Apple should be cut into quarters, the core removed and then chopped.
2. In a mid-sized bowl, combine all salad components except tuna.
3. Gently mix in the tuna.
4. Tuna apple salad can be used to stuff sandwiches that you make using lettuce and even whole bread that has been toasted if preferred.

Nutrition Facts Calories: 210 calories, Proteins: 37g, Carbs:11 g, Fat: 2g

5.6: Whole-wheat Broccoli Pasta

Prep Time: 30 minutes

Cook Time: 35 minutes

Servings: 1

Difficulty level: Easy

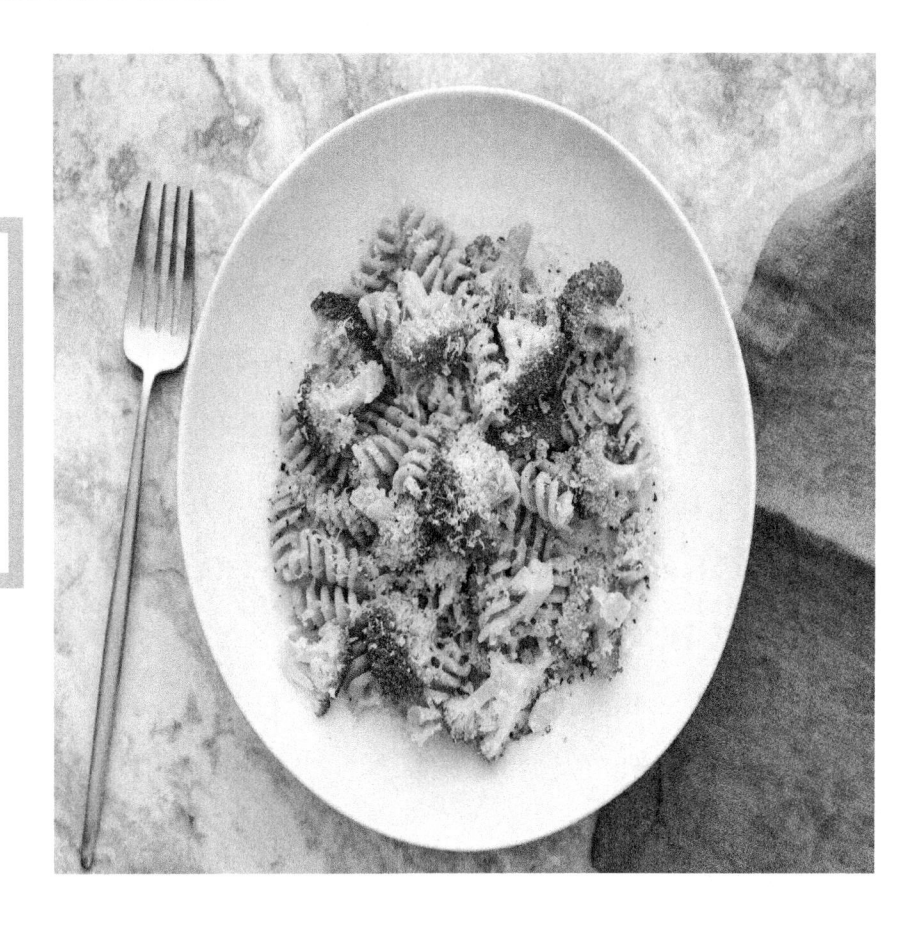

Ingredients

1/2 cup blanched broccoli florets	1/2 cup blanched carrot strips
salt and freshly ground black pepper	1/2 cup sliced onions
2 tsp olive oil	3 tbsp grated processed cheese
1/4 cup almonds	

Instructions

1. Start the boiling process with a large saucepan of water. Add the pasta, and cook it until it's al dente.
2. Drain, setting aside a half cup of the cooking liquid. Set aside.
3. Almonds should be crushed in a spice grinder until they become powdery.

4. After adding half of the lemon zest, some lemon juice, cloves, herbs, and a half teaspoon of salt, chop the ingredients in a food processor until they are outstanding. While the machine is running, slowly add the cooking water and oil and process until a smooth consistency is reached. Set pesto aside.

5. Mix the sauce in a large sauté pan over medium-high heat.

6. Apply a coating of cooking spray. Add the broccoli, pepper, and the extra 1 1/2 teaspoons of salt; continuing in batches, if necessary, sauté the broccoli, tossing it regularly, until it is lightly golden and crisp, which should take between 5 and 7 minutes.

7. Toss the pasta with the pesto. Once added — split it among 6 bowls.

8. Ricotta should be spread over the top, and the remaining zest should be sprinkled uniformly. Pour lemon juice over the topping.

9. Sometime before presenting, sprinkle the almond mixture that was sautéed earlier but was already left aside.

10. After planting, add a few extra virgin olive oil drops if the pasta lacks moisture. Immediately serve after cooking.

Nutrition Facts	Calories: 340 calories, Proteins: 25g, Carbs:12 g, Fat: 4g

5.7: Keto Enchidilas

Prep Time: 30 minutes

Cook Time: 45 minutes

Servings: 1

Difficulty level: Difficult

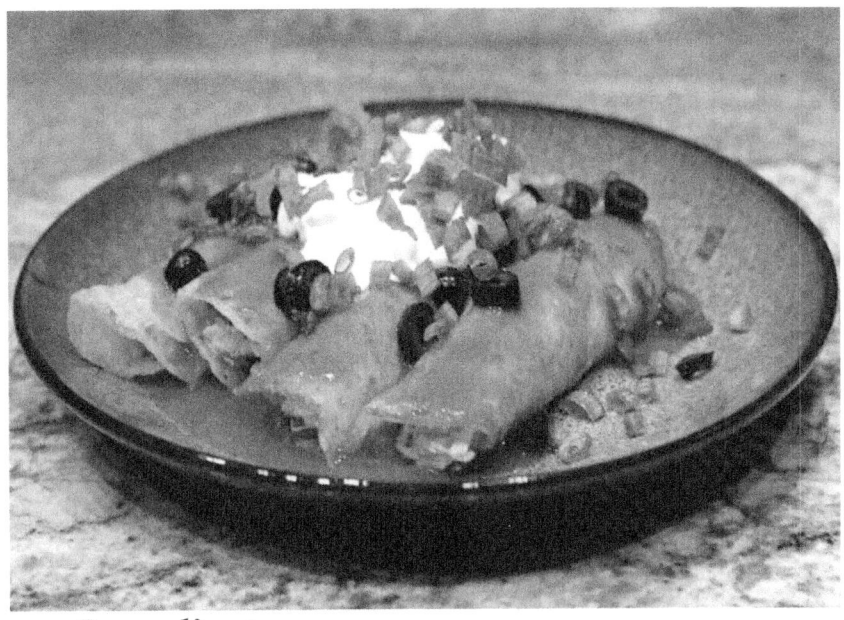

Ingredients

1 cremini wrap	2 tablespoons Mexican crema
2 ounces dried guajillo peppers	2 tablespoons tomatillo sauce
1 1/4 cups hot water or chicken broth	3 cloves garlic
2 tablespoons chopped cilantro	

Instructions

1. Heat a comal, hefty nonstick pan or cast-iron skillet to high temperatures and roast your peppers. Since you'll be dry roasting, the skillet should not have any oil added to it.
2. To roast your peppers, lay them in a pan over a heat source ranging from low to medium and toast each side of the peppers for one to two minutes. When they have reached the desired level of aroma, you will know they are ready. Be wary not to overdo them, as this might cause them to taste bitter.
3. The next step is to add the plum tomato slices, quartered onion, and unpeeled garlic cloves to the pan and then roast them until they are gently browned.
4. Trim the stems first from peppers and cut them in half while wearing gloves to protect your hands. Get rid of all of the seeds. If you want a sauce that is not as spicy, you should remove the skins because they contain heat.
5. Please put all of the peppers in a large basin and try pouring chicken or vegetable broth over them. Cover the bowl and let the peppers soak for about 25 seconds or until they grow pliable.
6. Put the peppers, roasted tomatoes, onion, garlic, and the liquid the peppers were soaking in into a

blender. Blend all of the ingredients until they are completely smooth and combined.

7. After the liquid has been blended to a smooth consistency, it is time to cook the sauce.

8. Prepare a pan with a capacity of 4 quarts by heating it over a medium flame and adding roughly a teaspoon of vegetable oil. After the oil has reached the desired temperature, add the chili and continue cooking over low heat, uncovered, until it reaches a boil. Before turning the heat, put it to a low simmer for approximately ten to fifteen minutes.

9. The recipe yields around 4-5 ounces and can be prepared in advance without problems. If frozen, the sauce can be saved for up to two weeks in the refrigerator and up to two months in the freezer. It is best to freeze the mixture in sections of one cup, as this will allow you to defrost only the amount needed. To make this chicken enchilada, you will only need to use one-half of the recipe. Because of this, you will have some sauce left over that you may use in other dishes.

10. To create these enchiladas, you will need two pounds of chicken thighs that have already been cooked and then seasoned with salt pepper, garlic powder, cumin concealer, and garlic powder. It also works very well with shredded chicken cooked in a rotisserie.

11. Putting together the enchiladas with chicken: Place a couple of teaspoons of enchilada sauce in the bottom of a baking dish 9 by 13 inches.

12. Establish a production line with the components of the Crepini thins, chile salsa, shredded chicken, and grated parmesan. Put approximately half of the enchilada sauce mixture into a bowl about the size of a medium bowl.

13. After dipping each wrap individually into the sauce, place approximately two spoonfuls of chicken into the center of each wrap and then roll it up. After that, sprinkle around two teaspoons of shredded cheese over the top. Wrap it up like a burrito and place it in the baking dish that's 9 by 13 inches.

14. Good, turn the stove temperature up to 350 degrees.

15. Continue doing this step by step until all the enchiladas have been assembled. The remaining sauce in the bowl should be poured over the enchiladas at this point. Bake for approximately 20–25 minutes after topping with the remaining amount of shredded cheese.

16. After the enchiladas have finished baking, top them with avocado chili, Mexican crema, and fresh cilantro that has been chopped.

17. The leftovers can be kept in an air-tight container for about three days or frozen for up to three weeks.

18. This recipe yields four and a half cups of enchilada sauce. You may go for a low-carb dieting enchilada sauce like Rosaria Enchilada Sauce if you're looking for a speedier alternative (2 cans).

Nutrition Facts   Calories: 340 calories, Proteins: 25g, Carbs:12 g, Fat: 4g

5.8: White Chicken

Prep Time: 30 minutes

Cook Time: 30 minutes

Servings: 1

Difficulty level: Easy

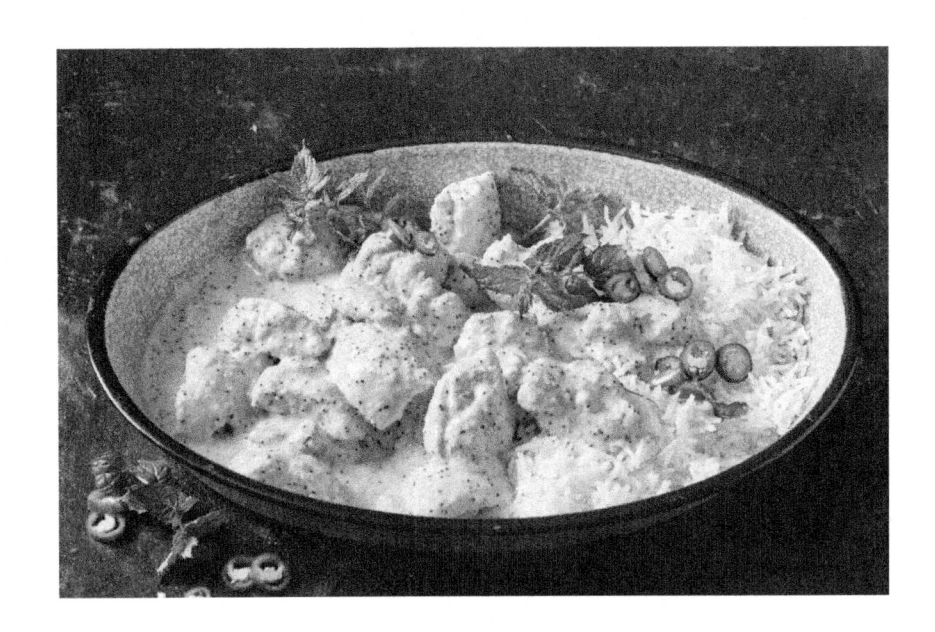

Ingredients

1/2 tsp cumin

2 tablespoons chopped cilantro

1/2 cup white beans

1/2 tsp Tabasco sauce

1/2 small white onion

1/4 cup shredded 2% cheddar cheese

1/2 lb boneless chicken breast

1 tablespoon light Italian dressing

1/2 can of green chilies

2 tablespoons plain Greek yogurt

1/2 can of chicken broth

Instructions

1. Bring the dressing to temperature in a large saucepan set over medium-high heat. After adding the chicken and onions, cook everything until the chicken is done. Mix it up every so often. *At this point, the dish can be moved to a slow cooker to be served later. Cook on low heat for 4-6 hours after adding the remaining ingredients.

2. Mix in the canned beans, broth, chilies, cumin, & tabasco sauce until well combined. Transport to a boil, then decrease the heat to a simmer and cook for ten minutes.

3. To serve, top with the following toppings: chopped cilantro, plain Greek yogurt, and shredded 2% cheddar cheese.

Nutrition Fact   Calories: 250 calories, Proteins: 23g, Carbs: 34g, Fat: 3g

Chapter 6: Dessert and Smoothie Recipes

6.1: Blueberry Cupcakes Lemon Icing

Prep Time: 15 minutes

Cook Time: 15 minutes

Servings: 1

Difficulty level: Moderate

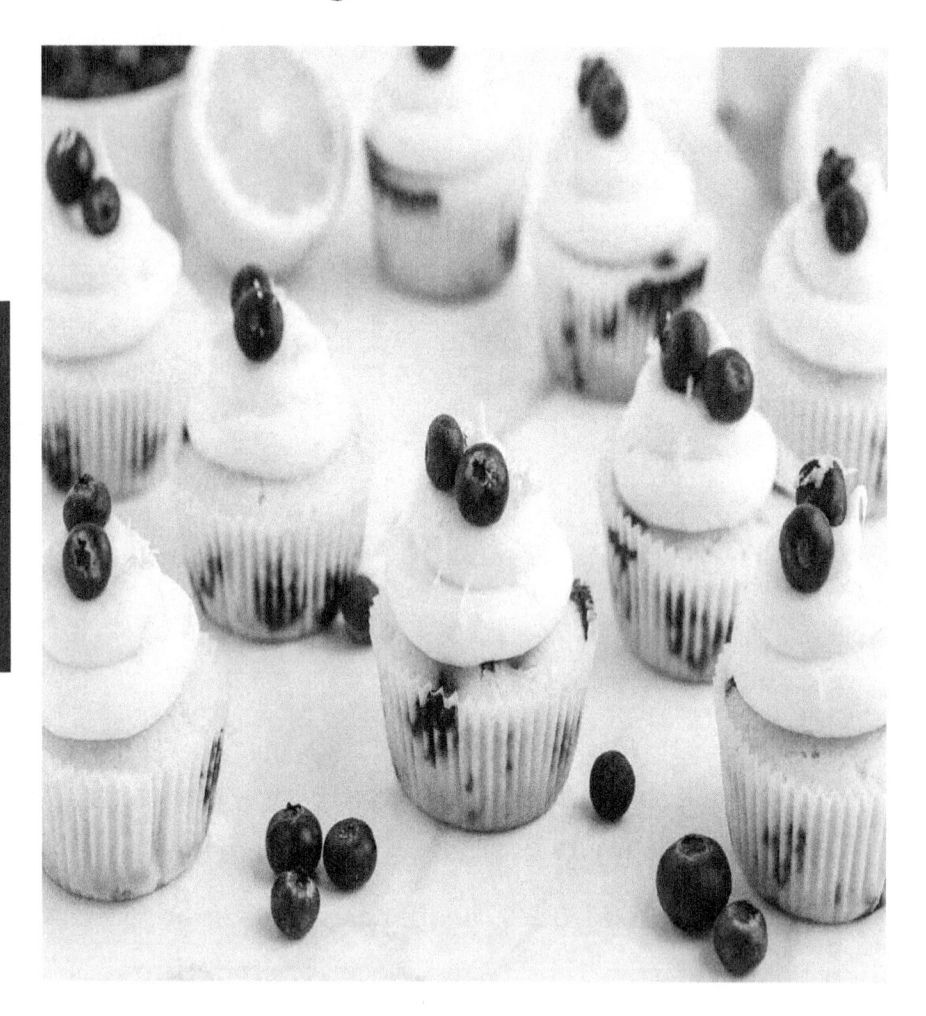

Ingredients

1/4 tsp Vanilla Extract	1 Chicken Egg
1 tbsp Lemon Juice	27.5 g Free Dairy Spread
27.5 g Self Raising Gluten Free Flour	Approx. 1/2 handful of Blueberries
112.5 g Icing Sugar	1/2 tsp Coconut Milk
27.5 g Sugar	

Instructions

1. Raise the temperature of the microwave to 180 degrees Celsius before using it (350F)

2. Blend or mix the dairy-free spread and sugar for several minutes using either a hand mixer or a blender.

3. In a bowl, mix the eggs by whisking them with a metal fork. Mix the contents of one egg spoon with one tablespoon of flour into the combination of melted butter and sugar. Do this for a few seconds. After that, combine another level teaspoonful of egg and flour until the whole egg has been worked in. Through the use of this procedure, the mixture will not get curdled. Incorporate any remaining flour and thoroughly mix it.

4. Mix for a few seconds after adding fresh coconut milk and vanilla essence.

5. Include the blueberries and mix them by hand after adding them.

6. After distributing the mixture equally among the 12 cupcake liners, place the batter in the saucepan for ten to fifteen minutes. When done, they should have a hue similar to a golden brown and a bouncy texture.

7. When adding the frosting, add the lemon juice to a container such as a bowl, and while mixing, sift the powdered sugar into the bowl. Keep adding more icing sugar until you get a consistency that is thick and resistant to dripping.

8. After the cakes have had time to cool, you may frost them and then place a blueberry on top of the frosting on each cake. Put the cakes in the refrigerator so that the icing can be set.

| **Nutrition Facts** | Calories: 271 calories, Proteins: 4g, Carbs: 24g, Fat: 18g |

6.2: Carrot Cake

Prep Time: 10 minutes

Cook Time: 40 minutes

Servings: 1

Difficulty level: Difficult

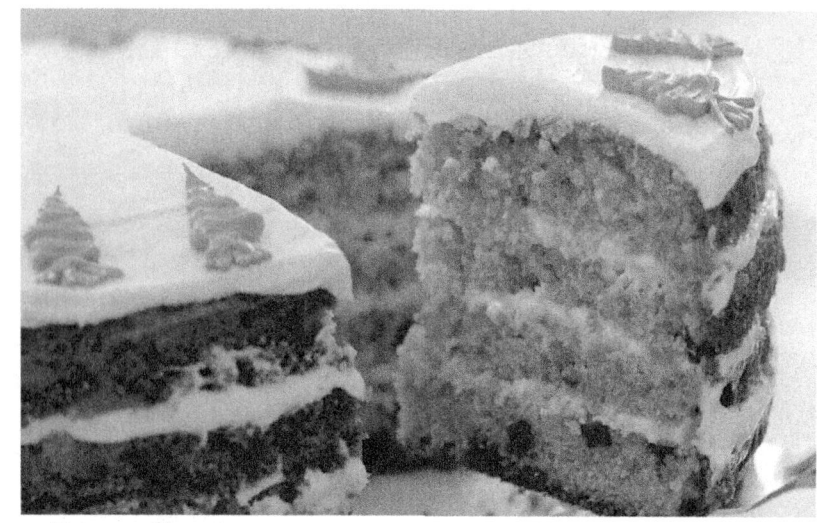

Ingredients

45g Sugar, Caster	1 Chicken Egg
62.5g grated Carrots	45ml Vegetable Oil
50g Icing Sugar	40g Plain Flour
1/2 tsp Bicarbonate of Soda	1/4 tsp Cinnamon, ground
6.25g Spread	15g Walnuts (optional)
50g Cream Cheese	

Instructions

1. Preheat the oven to 160 degrees Celsius.
2. When I grease a cake pan, I turn to dairy-free margarine. This cake has the perfect proportions to fit into a loaf pan.
3. A mixing bowl should fully incorporate all of the cake's components except the carrots and walnuts.
4. After adding the carrots to the mixture, ensure they are properly mixed.
5. Baking the batter in the oven for about 1 hour and five minutes, or until a knife implanted/inserted into the middle of the cake comes out clean, is recommended.
6. After that, make the frosting by beating together dairy-free spread, dairy-free cream cheese, and icing sugar in a mixer until smooth. When you don't want the frosting to have an overpowering sweetness, reduce the quantity of icing sugar you use.
7. When the cake has reached the desired temperature, the frosting may be applied to the top. This ganache does not include any dairy; thus, it is quite runny.

Nutrition Facts Calories: 390 calories, Proteins: 7.8g, Carbs: 14.4g, Fat: 35.7g

6.3: Apple Chunks Oatmeal Cookies

Prep Time: 15 minutes

Cook Time: 45 minutes

Servings: 1

Difficulty level: Intermediate

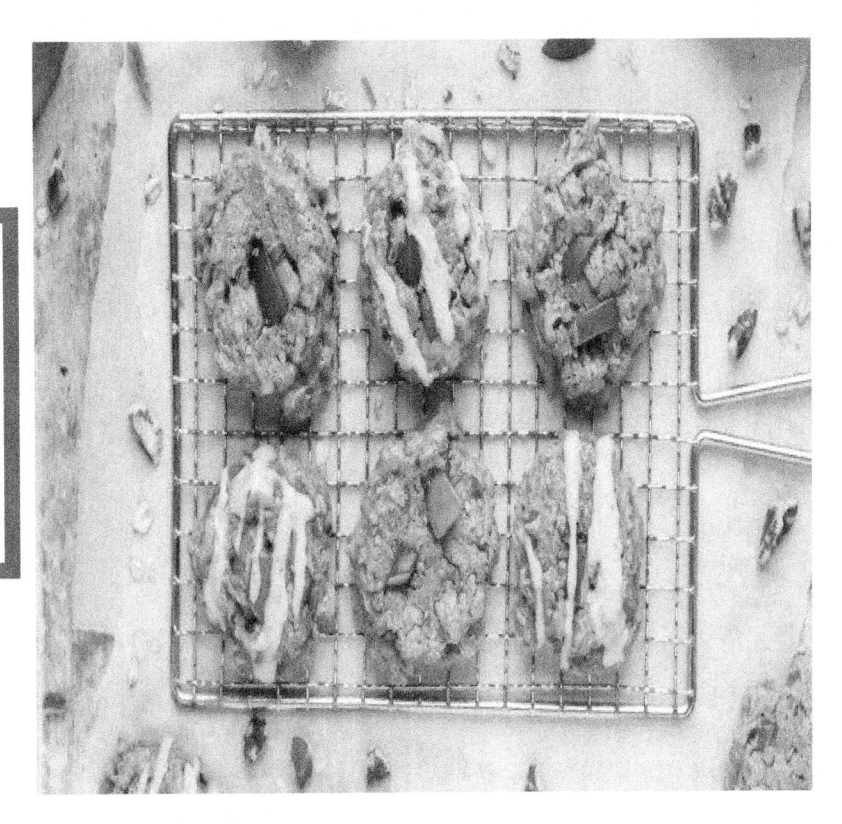

Ingredients

1/4 cup coarsely shredded and peeled apple	1/8 tsp salt
1/4 tsp vanilla extract	1/16 tsp ground nutmeg
1 large egg white or 2 tsp dry egg whites	1/8 tsp baking powder
1/4 cup diced dried apples	1/4 tsp baking soda
1/2 cup old-fashioned oats	1/4 tsp ground cinnamon
1/4 cup chopped walnuts	2 tbsp granulated sugar
1 tbsp canola oil	

Instructions

1. To get the oven ready, heat it to 375 degrees Fahrenheit.

2. The oats and the nuts should be spread out in a single coating/layer on a baking sheet.

3. After baking until fragrant and browned, remove from the oven and set aside for five to ten minutes.

4. Prepare two baking sheets by coating them with cooking spray and setting them aside.

5. Whole-wheat pastry flour is a kind of flour that may be found at health food shops. This flour gives baked goods a light texture while also providing fiber.

6. Put the container, which should be airtight, into the refrigerator or the freezer.

7. Mix the egg whites, apple shreds, butter, granulated sugar, brown sugar oil, and vanilla essence in a large bowl. Use a spoon to stir the concoction until all ingredients are evenly distributed.

8. After adding the dry ingredients, mix the wet and dry components until the dry component is almost completely dry. Combine the dried apples with the oats, almonds, and other saved ingredients.

9. Put the dough on the baking sheets prepared by level tablespoonfuls, being sure to leave about 2 inches of space in the center of each one.

10. Mix the remaining 1 tablespoon of granulated sugar and 1/4 teaspoon of cinnamon in a separate dish using the smaller bowl. Spray some cooking spray onto the bottom of the glass where it will sit.

11. After being initially submerged in the cinnamon sugar, the cookies should be pressed down with the glass, which should be repeated for each cookie.

12. It should take between 010 and 012 minutes, depending on the size of the cookie sheet, to bake until they have a color between golden and light brown. It is best practice to wrap food in plastic and then in foil before placing it in the freezer for an extended period. When storing food in the freezer for an extended period, it is best to practice waiting two minutes for the cookies to cool completely on the baking pans before transferring them to wire racks. The plastic will help to avoid freezer burn, and the foil will prevent unpleasant aromas from reaching the food. The double layer of protection provides both benefits.

Nutrition Facts Calories: 66 calories, Proteins: 1.1g, Carbs: 10.8g, Fat: 2.1g

6.4: Chocolate Cake

Prep Time: 15 minutes

Cook Time: 50 minutes

Servings: 1

Difficulty level: Intermediate

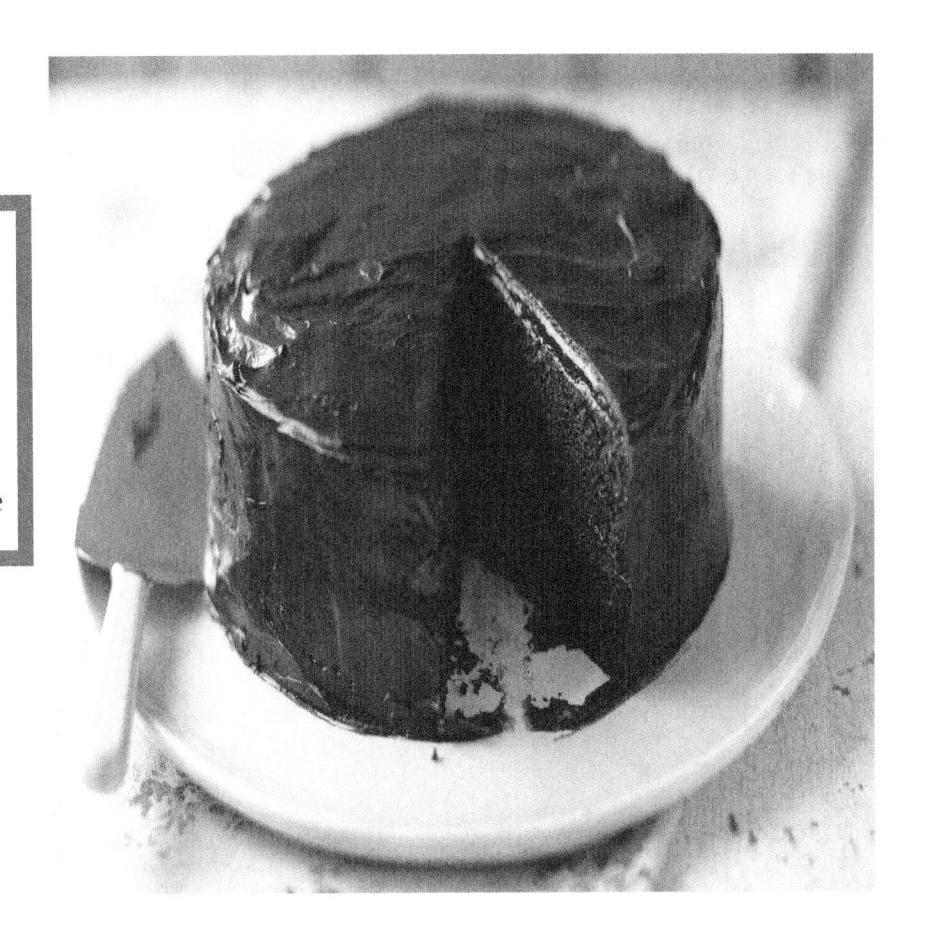

Ingredients

Granulated sugar for dusting (as needed)	1 tbsp canola oil
2 tbsp unsweetened cocoa powder	1/4 cup packed brown sugar
1/2 tsp vanilla extract	1 lightly beaten egg
1/4 cup of hot black coffee	1 cup whole-wheat flour
1/4 cup granulated sugar	(Pastry flour can be used)
A pinch of salt	1/2 tsp baking powder
1/2 tsp baking soda	

Instructions

1. The temperature in the oven should be raised to 350 degrees Fahrenheit.
2. Spray some cooking spray into a round cake pan with a diameter of 9 inches.
3. Place a piece of parchment paper cut into a circle at the bottom of the pan.
4. Mix and whisk together all ingredients in a large basin, including granulated sugar, baking powder, cocoa powder, baking soda, and salt. Whole-wheat flour should also be included in this step. Whole-wheat pastry flour is a wonderful choice for generating softer baked goods since it has a lower potential to produce gluten and has less protein than traditional whole-wheat flour. Additionally, whole-wheat pastry flour is used in fewer recipes. These may be found in the natural foods section of grocery shops and establishments specifically devoted to selling natural foods. Place in the refrigerator to prevent spoilage.
5. Mix some buttermilk, brown sugar, oil, and vanilla extract with an egg. If you cannot get buttermilk, you may use buttermilk powder instead of the liquid form of buttermilk and combine it per the directions provided with the recipe. A similar effect may be achieved by combining one tablespoon of lemon juice with one cup of milk and swirling the concoction. You could also use vinegar instead of lemon; you might try sour or sour milk.
6. Mixing using a mixer on a somewhat high speed for two minutes is recommended.
7. While using a beater, incorporate the heated coffee into the batter. It will result in the batter having a more liquid consistency.
8. The mixture should be poured into the dish that has already been prepared.
9. Bake the cake for thirty-five to forty-five minutes, checking it every five minutes to ensure that a skewer incorporated/inserted into the center comes out clean.
10. After taking the cake from the pan and letting it rest for ten minutes on a rack inside the refrigerator, it is now time to take it from the pan, remove all the wax paper from the pan, and then allow the cake to cool completely before serving.
11. Sprinkle confectioners' sugar over it just before cutting it into pieces.

Nutrition Facts	Calories: 139calories, Proteins: 2.3g, Carbs: 26.6g, Fat: 3.2g

6.5: Pear and Ginger smoothie

Prep Time: 2 minutes

Cook Time: 5 minutes

Servings: 1

Difficulty level: Easy

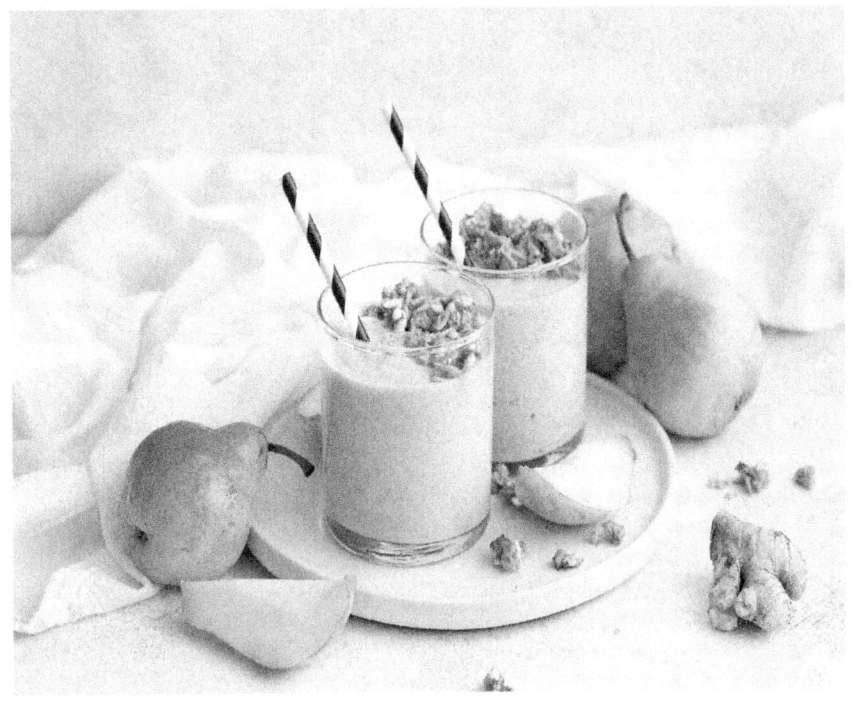

Ingredients

300ml Water approx.	1 Apple
Ginger fresh, small piece	1 Pear ripe

Instructions

1. Both the pear and the apple should have their stems and cores removed.
2. Reduced to little pieces
3. Please take out a handful of fresh ginger, around the size of a pound coin, and put it away in a separate bowl.
4. Put everything in your blender, fill it to the top with filtered water, and give it a whirl for a quarter of a minute.
5. Enjoy!

Nutrition Facts   Calories: 80 calories, Proteins: 1g, Carbs: 18g, Fat: 6g

6.6: Mixed Berry Smoothie

Prep Time: 5 minutes

Cook Time: 0 minutes

Servings: 1

Difficulty level: Easy

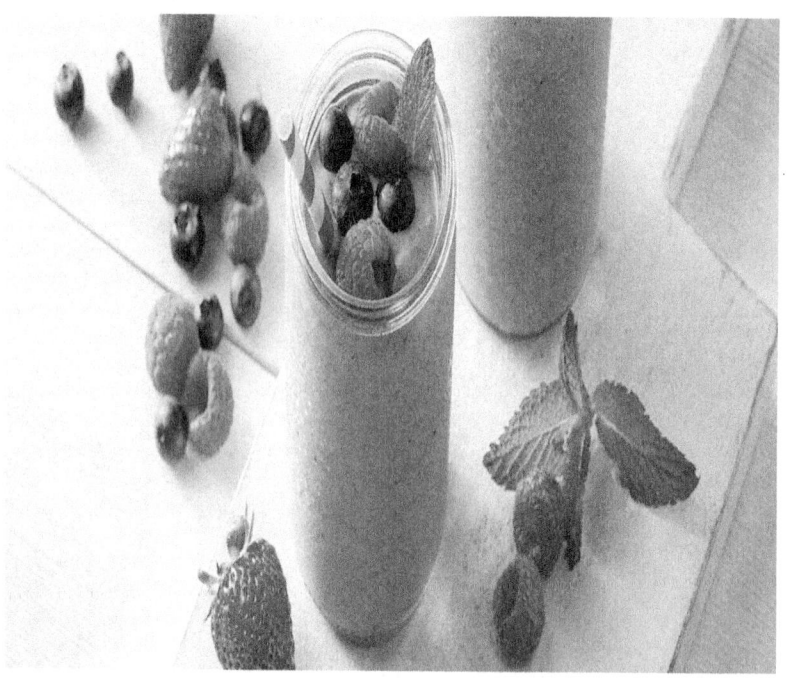

Ingredients

3/4 cup mixed berries	1/2 cup Greek yogurt
1/2 cup liquid of choice	1/2 sliced banana
1/2 tbsp honey	1 tbsp oats

Instructions

1. Put some frozen fruit, a banana, some yogurt, some oats, and whichever liquid you like most into the jug of your blender. Blend until smooth. Combine until there are no lumps.

2. Blend it up until it's as smooth as silk, and then, if required, add more liquid and mix it again.

3. After you have sampled the smoothie, quickly add as much honey as you like and blend it.

4. After you have poured the mixture into glasses, you may garnish them with fresh berries.

5. If you use a powdered blender with a lot of power, adding a tablespoon or more flax or chia seeds to your drink can provide you with an additional supply of omega-3 fatty acids.

6. You might try mixing frozen or fresh spinach or kale to increase the smoothie's nutritional content. Don't make it extremely sweet!

7. If the beverage of your choice is apple or grape juice, you are not advised to add honey in the preparation of the beverage.

8. Add More Fruit, and if you want to give the smoothie a more out-of-the-ordinary twist, try mixing in some frozen pieces of mango or pineapple.

9. You might use a banana that has been frozen in its place if you have one available to you.

10. You can experiment with your smoothie in any way you see fit; feel free to add pure vanilla essence, powdered ginger, or anything else you enjoy that pairs deliciously with the berry's flavor.

| **Nutrition Facts** | Calories: 150 calories, Proteins: 5.5g, Carbs: 20g, Fat: 0.2g |

6.7: Orange Smoothie

Prep Time: 5 minutes

Cook Time: 0 minutes

Servings: 1

Difficulty level: Easy

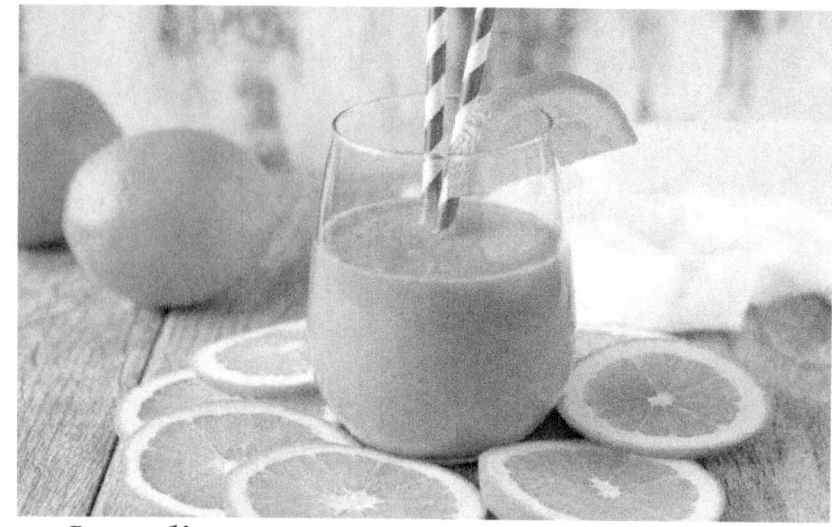

Ingredients

1 tsp Nature Nate's honey	1/2 frozen banana
1/4 tsp vanilla extract	1/4 cup plain Greek yogurt
1/4 cup unsweetened oat milk	1 cup frozen blood orange wedges

Instructions

1. To get the blood oranges ready for freezing, peel them and remove any seeds that may be within. When you have finished separating the wedges, please place them in a particular layer on a baking sheet that has been previously prepared.
2. Please make sure the baking sheet has been chilled for some time in the refrigerator before using it. Kindly move it to a location where it may be flat.
3. Put the wedges in the freezer for about two hours or until they have reached an entirely frozen condition.
4. You can put the wedges in a bag or use them in the smoothie.
5. Put the blood oranges that have been frozen into a food processor or a blender, and then mix them with the remaining ingredients. Combine until there are no lumps!
6. Other components, such as shredded hemp flakes, flax hearts, milled flax, ground flax, chia seeds, almond butter, or frozen fruit, might also be included.
7. If you want to make this smoothie, you have up to a day's head start on getting started. The food should be refrigerated in a container that can completely exclude air.

Nutrition Facts Calories: 340 calories, Proteins: 9.9g, Carbs: 27g, Fat: 1.0g.

6.8: Dragon Fruit Smoothie

Prep Time: 5 minutes

Cook Time: 1 minute

Servings: 1

Difficulty Level: Easy

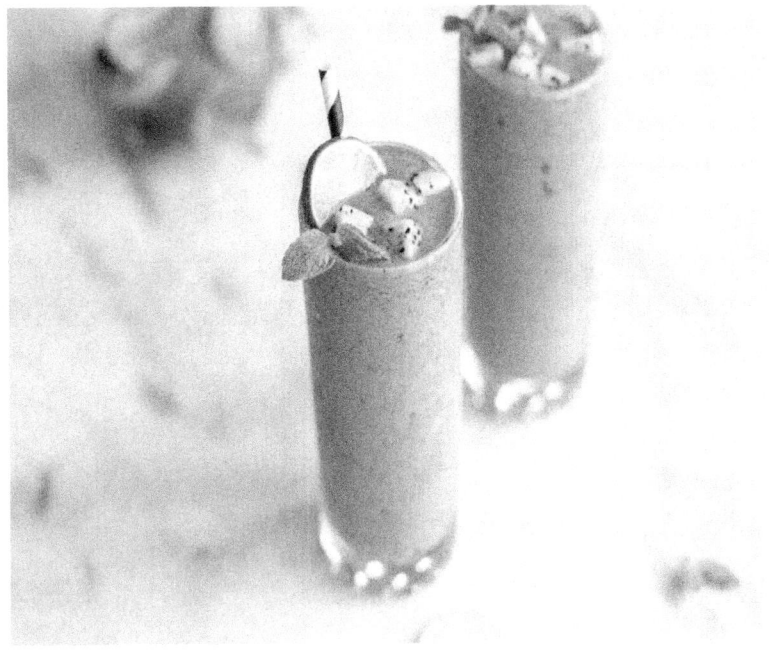

Ingredients

1/2 cup raspberries	1/4 – 1/2 cup milk
3 Tbsp Vanilla Protein Powder	2 packets of dragon fruit
2 ripe bananas	

Instructions

1. A powerful blender combines frozen fruit, raspberry, banana, whey protein, and dairy-free milk into a smoothie. The secret to making a bowl of thick smoothies is to be patient and blend the ingredients gently while simultaneously adding as much liquid as is necessary and scraping the sides of the container with a smoothie wand (or something else that is safe to use in a blender) while the mixture is being blended.

2. To serve, top with toppings like fruit, granola, hemp oil, and coconut flakes (optional).

3. When it's feasible, serve the food right away. The leftovers may be stored in the fridge-freezer for up to 024 hours after they have been prepared. Freeze it to make it last for a longer period. Another option is to freeze the fruit in ice cube trays to be used later in smoothies.

Nutrition Facts	Calories: 225 calories, Proteins: 8g, Carbs: 48g, Fat: 2g.

6.9: Peanut Butter Banana Porridge

Prep Time: 10 minutes

Cook Time: 15 minutes

Servings: 1

Difficulty level: Easy

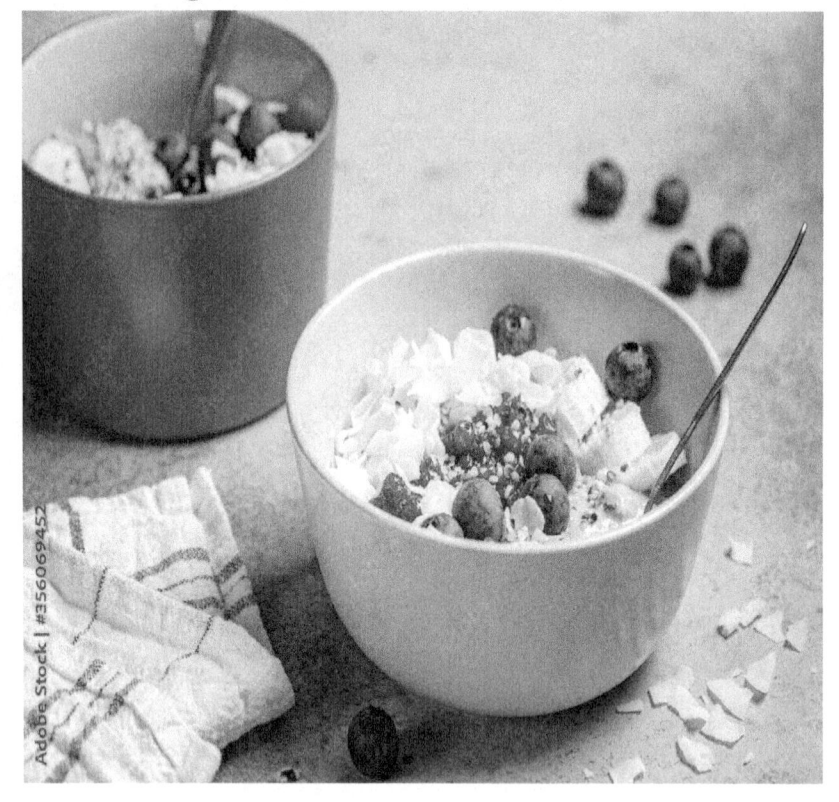

Ingredients

1/2 cup old-fashioned oats	Optional: 1 scoop of protein powder
1 cup water	Pinch of salt
1 medium banana, mashed	1 tsp. vanilla extract
1 tbsp. peanut butter	1 tsp. honey

Instructions

1. Bring the tap/mineral water to a boil in a saucepan of a manageable size.
2. Mix the oats, salt, and vanilla essence using a stirring motion.
3. Reduce the heat, and cook the oats over a low simmer for about five to seven minutes, stirring the mixture regularly.
4. Mix the honey, peanut butter, and mashed bananas using a wooden spoon.
5. Enjoy while it's still hot!

Nutrition Facts   Calories: 360 calories, Proteins: 10g, Carbs: 62g, Fat: 12g

6.10: Creamy Rice Porridge

Prep Time: 15 minutes

Cook Time: 10 minutes

Servings: 1

Difficulty level: Easy

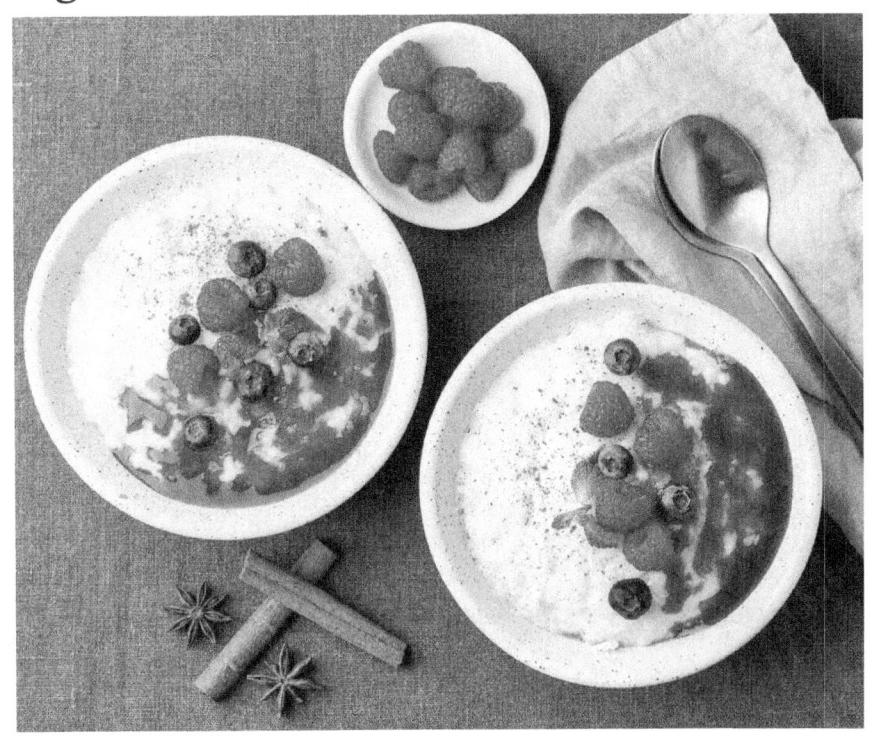

Ingredients

1 cup of plain old rice

2 ounces of water

half a cup of heavy cream

1/4 milligram of salt 1/4 cup of honey

or your preferred sweetness

Instructions

1. The white rice, water, heavy cream, and salt should all be combined in a medium-sized pot.
2. Bring the combination to a boil, then decrease the heat and let it simmer for 018 to 020 minutes or until the rice is soft and creamy.
3. Mix in the honey or whatever sweetener you like.
4. Serve and enjoy

Nutrition Facts   Calories: 348 calories, Proteins: 8g, Carbs: 53g, Fat: 12g

Chapter 7: Dinner Recipes

7.1: Meatloaf Muffins with Barbecue

Prep Time: 15 minutes

Cook Time: 40 minutes

Servings: 1

Difficulty level: Easy

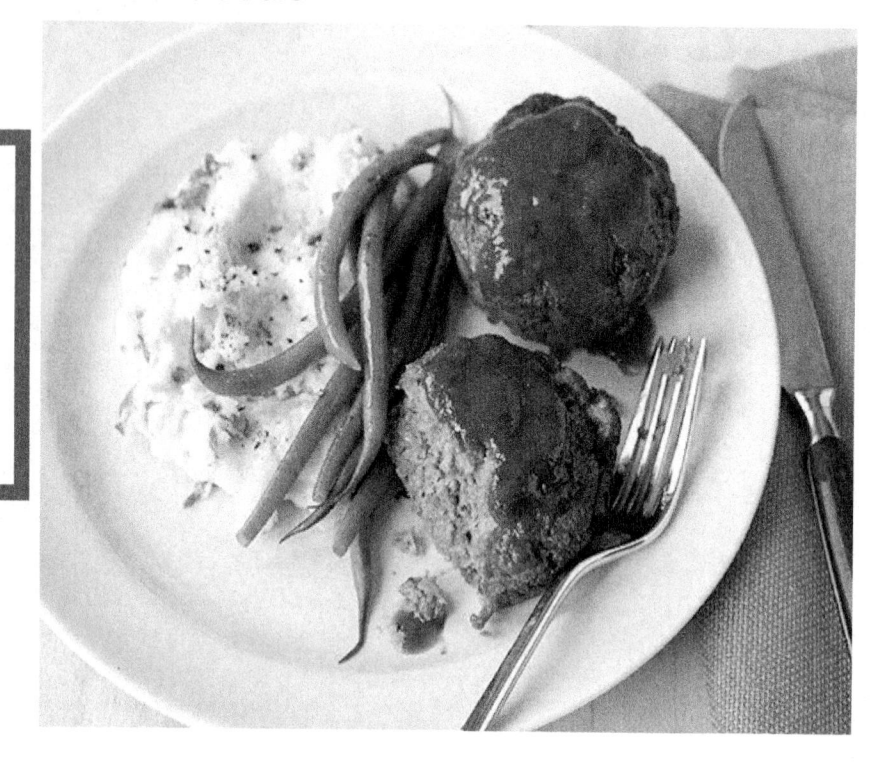

Ingredients

1 slice multigrain bread	2 tbsp barbecue sauce
Fresh pepper	1 egg
2 tbsp barbecue sauce	1/2 cup onions
1/8 tsp salt	1/2 package of ground turkey breast
1 tbsp Worcestershire sauce	

Instructions

1. Raise the temperature in the oven to 350 degrees Fahrenheit. Apply culinary spray inside a regular muffin tray with 12 separate cups. Because this recipe makes nine meatloaf muffins, you only need to fill nine rather than all twelve. Set aside.

2. A slice of bread baked with whole or several grains was toasted. Place in a mixer and process until the consistency of bread crumbs is reached.

3. Thoroughly combine the ground turkey, croutons, onions, egg, Sauce, and a quarter cup of barbecue sauce in a large bowl. Mix until everything is evenly distributed. Add little salt and Pepper before serving. To properly blend the ingredients, use your fingers or a large spoon until they are incorporated.

4. Evenly distribute the meatloaf mixture over the tops of the nine muffin cups that have been prepped. On top of each meatloaf muffin, place three-quarters of a teaspoon's worth of barbecue sauce and spread it out so it's fairly distributed.

5. Bake for about 40 minutes. Run a knife across the outside of every muffin to remove it from the pan. Place the meat on a serving dish when you have transferred it.

| **Nutrition Facts** | Calories: 115 calories, Proteins: 18g, Carbs: 18g, Fat: 2g |

7.2: Chicken Fajita Bowls

Prep Time: 20 minutes

Cook Time: 30 minutes

Servings: 1

Difficulty level: Easy

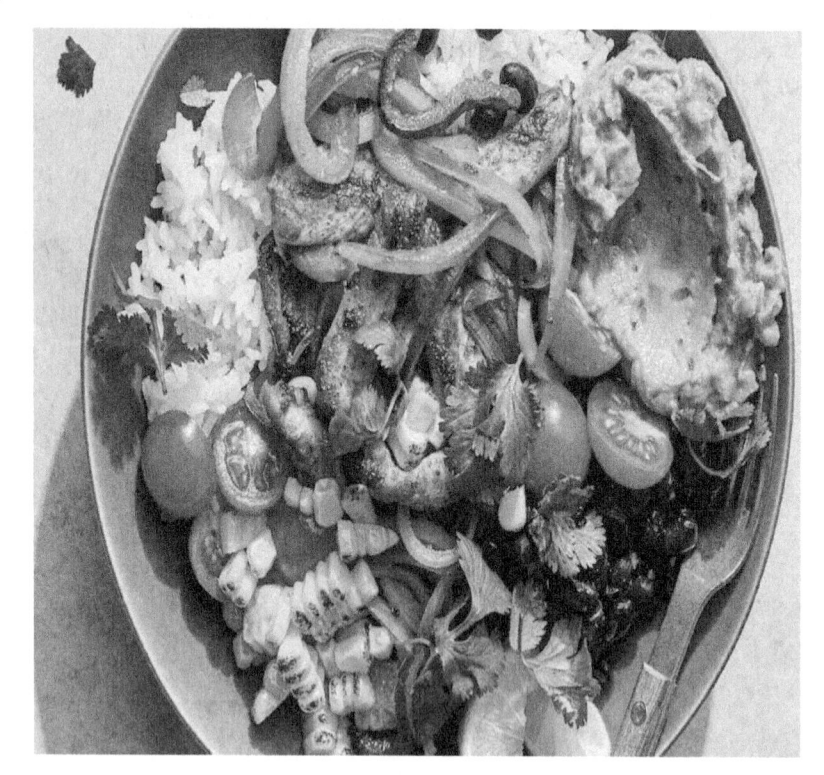

Ingredients

1/2 tsp garlic salt	2 tbsp chopped cilantro
1/2 tsp cumin	1 tbsp tomato paste
Salt and pepper to taste	1/2 red bell pepper
1 tbsp avocado or olive oil	1/2 yellow bell pepper
1/2-3/4 lbs chicken breast	Juice of 1/4 lime
1/2 green bell pepper	1 tbsp avocado or olive oil
1/2 tsp garlic salt	Juice of 1/2 lime
2 cups riced cauliflower	Salt and pepper to taste
1/2 orange bell pepper	1/2 white onion
1/2 tsp garlic salt	1/4-1/2 tsp chipotle powder

Instructions

1. Put the ingredients again for chicken marinade, oil, lemon zest, chipotle powder, garlic powder, and tomato paste in a shallow dish. Mix the ingredients.

2. After patting the chicken breasts clean with a paper towel, place them inside a freezer bag with the marinade, then shake the bag to ensure that the marinade evenly coats the chicken. Set aside.

3. A pan is ready to be used after it has been heated at medium-high heat and then coated with cooking spray.

4. The cauliflower should be boiled until it is soft, then riced cauliflower, garlic powder, salt, and Pepper to preference should be added. Finally, the cauliflower must be cooked (about 5-7 minutes).

5. After mixing the cauliflower with lime juice and the chopped cilantro in a bowl, set the cauliflower mixture to the side.

6. While the pan is continuing to heat up, add the chopped onions and one oil tablespoon to the pan. Sauté for around 1-2 minutes

7. In a pan, sauté sliced red peppers with garlic salt and cumin for a sufficient amount of time so that the veggies are cooked throughout but still retain some of their crispness (about 4-5 minutes). Set aside.

8. If more oil is required, add it to the pan before frying the chicken for another 4-5 minutes per side (depending on its thickness) or until the chicken isn't any longer pink in the center.

9. Prepare bowls containing chicken, fajita vegetables, and rice made from cauliflower.

10. You may garnish it with lime, coriander, and avocado if you'd like, but doing so is completely optional.

| **Nutrition Facts** | Calories: 356 calories, Proteins: 42g, Carbs: 12g, Fat: 4g |

7.3: Garlic Butter Salmon

Prep Time: 10 minutes

Cook Time: 10 minutes

Servings: 1

Difficulty level: Easy

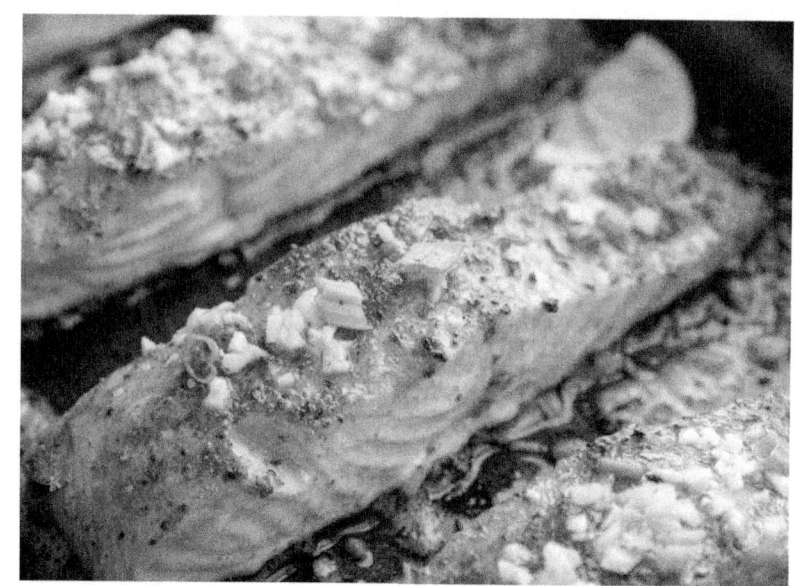

Ingredients

1 tsp olive oil	1/8 tsp salt
1/2 tsp Italian seasoning	3/4 lb salmon fillet
1 1/2 finely minced garlic cloves	Black pepper to taste
1 tbsp butter	1/4 lemon juice only

Instructions

1. Put the pizza dough in the oven and preheat it to 400 °. Place all the fish in a large baking dish with a rim that can easily contain it all (the cooking pan is there to catch any drippings; it'll be much easier to clean than your oven!). Bake the salmon according to the package directions. Wrap the baking sheet with a big layer of aluminum and place it in the oven.

2. The Best of the Season's Fish: Olive oil has to be used to gently grease the foil. Arrange the salmon fillets over the rest of the ingredients. First, drizzle the surface, including one tablespoon of oil, and then evenly disperse the garlic cloves over the top of the olive oil. Sprinkle with Italian seasonings, salt, and Pepper, and then finish by drizzling with lemon juice while continuing to season with Italian seasoning. Dot the surface with some butter — seal foil around the salmon.

3. Bake: Heat the stove to 350 degrees Fahrenheit, and bake your salmon fillets for ten to fifteen minutes, based on the thickness of the fillets, or until the fish easily separates into individual pieces. Serve at once after the cooking.

Nutrition Facts   Calories: 328 calories, Proteins: 34g, Carbs: 1g, Fat: 20g

7.4: Cauliflower Casserole

Prep Time: 10 minutes

Cook Time: 40 minutes

Servings: 1

Difficulty level: Easy

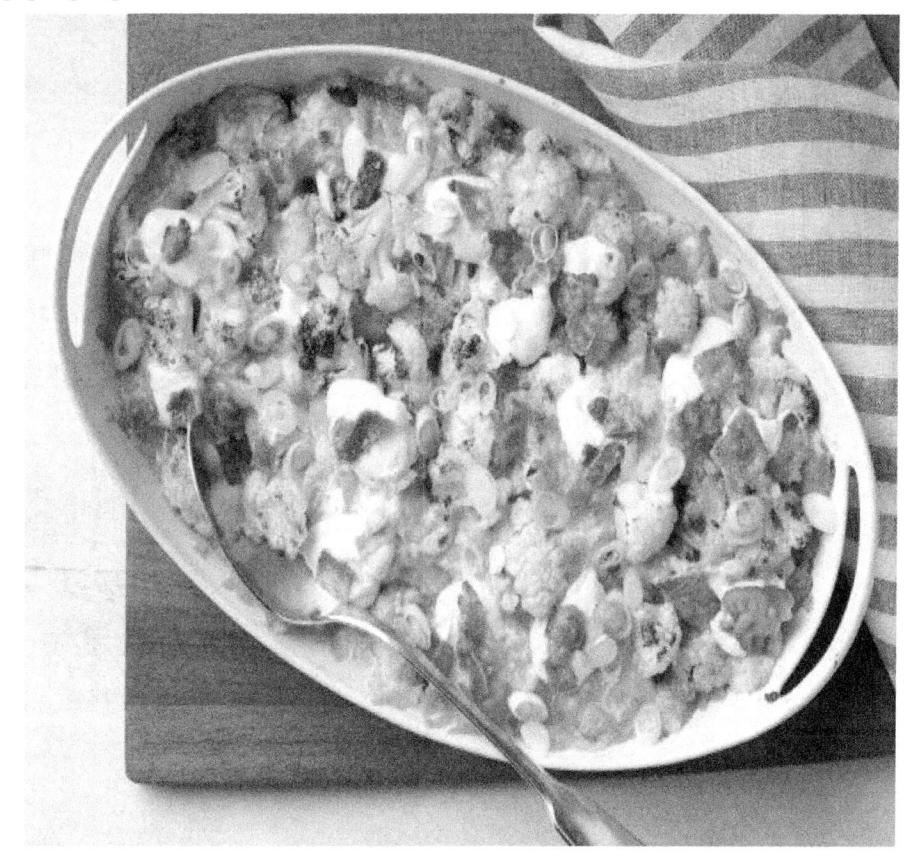

Ingredients

Salt and Pepper	¼ cup red Pepper
16 oz turkey sausage	1 cup ricotta cheese
1 clove garlic	2-4 cups steamed cauliflower
¼ cup onion	¼ cup broth
1-2 cups spinach	¼ cup mushrooms

Instructions

1. Prepare a saute pan with nonstick cooking spray and heat it over medium heat. Add turkey sausage and break it into bite-sized bits with a wooden spoon. Remove the fat.

2. After the sausage has cooked most of the way, stir in the onion, red Pepper, greens, and mushrooms, and season with Pepper and salt to taste. Saute for 3-30 mins or until veggies soften. After adding the garlic, stir it for a minute without letting it burn, and then add the broth. Please bring it to a boil, but immediately remove the pot from the heat.

3. Apply some nonstick spray to the inside of the casserole dish. After adding the cooked cauliflower and ricotta cheese, thoroughly combine the ingredients. The casserole dish should be topped with a mixture of meat and vegetables. Stir to mix.

4. Bake for 10 to 15 minutes in an oven preheated to 350 degrees. After adding the parmesan cheese, return the dish to the oven for another few minutes for the cheese to melt.

5. Ricotta or broth should provide moisture to this meal, which should assist patients who have had gastric sleeve, bariatric surgery, or lap band surgery to handle it better.

6. Cauliflower is a very flexible vegetable option. It can be included in flavor profiles, such as Italian, Asian, or Latino meals. It does so without contributing a great deal in the way of calories or carbs. In addition to a wide variety of vitamins and minerals, forty calories, three grams of fiber, eight grams of carbs, and three grams of protein are included inside a cup of cooked and fresh cauliflower florets.

Nutrition Facts   Calories: 328 calories, Proteins: 34g, Carbs: 1g, Fat: 20g

7.5: Bell Pepper Soup

Prep Time: 15 minutes

Cook Time: 35 minutes

Servings: 1

Difficulty level: Easy

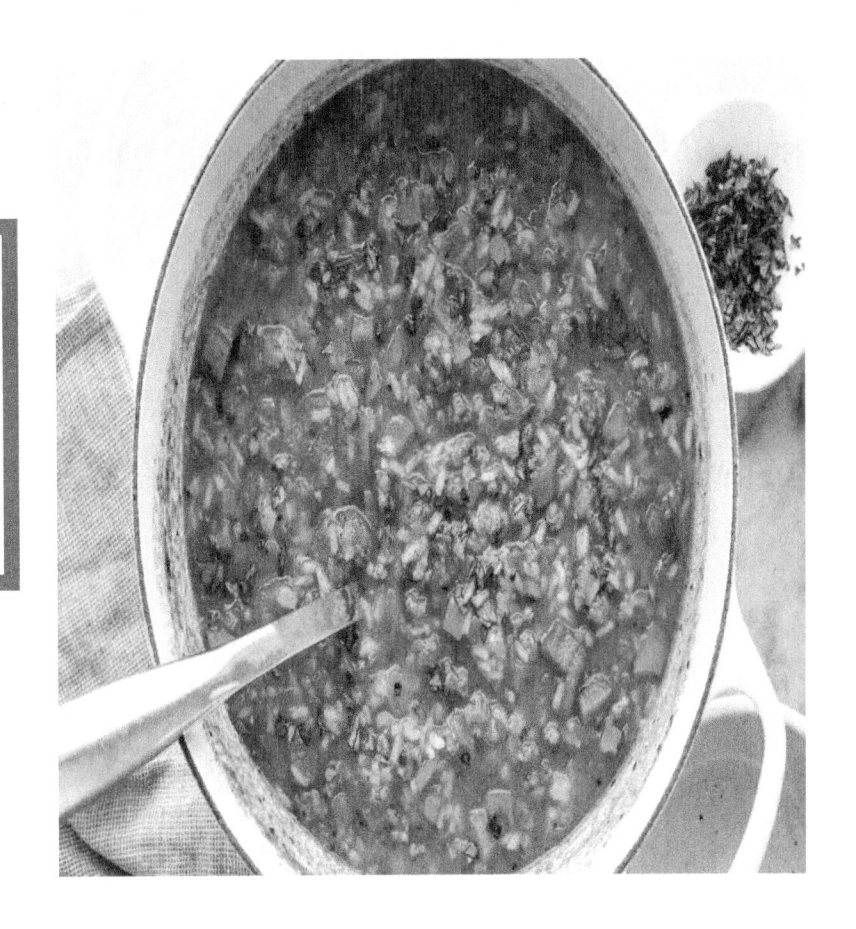

Ingredients

2 tbsp extra-virgin olive oil	1 1/2 tsp fresh marjoram
1 medium sweet potato	1 1/2 tsp Sensational Sriracha Sauce
Sea salt and ground black pepper to taste	1/4 small onion
1/4 cup chopped fresh cilantro	4 yellow and red bell peppers
2 cups vegetable broth	1/2 celery stalk
1 medium carrot	1 sliced avocado
1/2 recipe of Gluten-Free Herbed Croutons	

Instructions

1. To prepare the oil, heat it in a big saucepan above medium heat until it reaches the desired temperature. In addition to the sliced onion, carrot, and celery, you should also include a pinch of salt and a few grinds of black pepper. After four minutes of cooking, the vegetables should be soft enough to pierce with a fork.

2. When the onion has been cooking for about six minutes, add the red peppers and keep stirring them until they are soft.

3. Add the potatoes to the stock that already contains the sweet potatoes. The pot should be covered and then seasoned with salt or black pepper before being brought to a boil.

4. Then wait until the mixture reaches a full rolling boil. Bring the temperature down, then add the marjoram while stirring. Maintain a low simmer for approximately 20 minutes or until vegetables have the desired softness.

5. After allowing the stew to cool gradually, transfer portions to a blender and puree until it reaches a smooth consistency. If it's too sticky for your taste, you may thin it down by adding extra water. Salt or black pepper must be added to the dish to modify the seasoning. After returning the soup to the pot, keep it warm over a low flame until it is ready to serve. Croutons seasoned with herbs should be used as a decoration, along with avocado, coriander, and the Sensational Fajita Seasoning, if that is what the customer wants. It is recommended that the sauce be served on the side of the food.

Nutrition Facts	Calories: 172 calories, Proteins: 34g, Carbs: 1g, Fat: 20g

7.6: Chickpea Curry

Prep Time: 25 minutes

Cook Time: 30 minutes

Servings: 1

Difficulty level: Easy

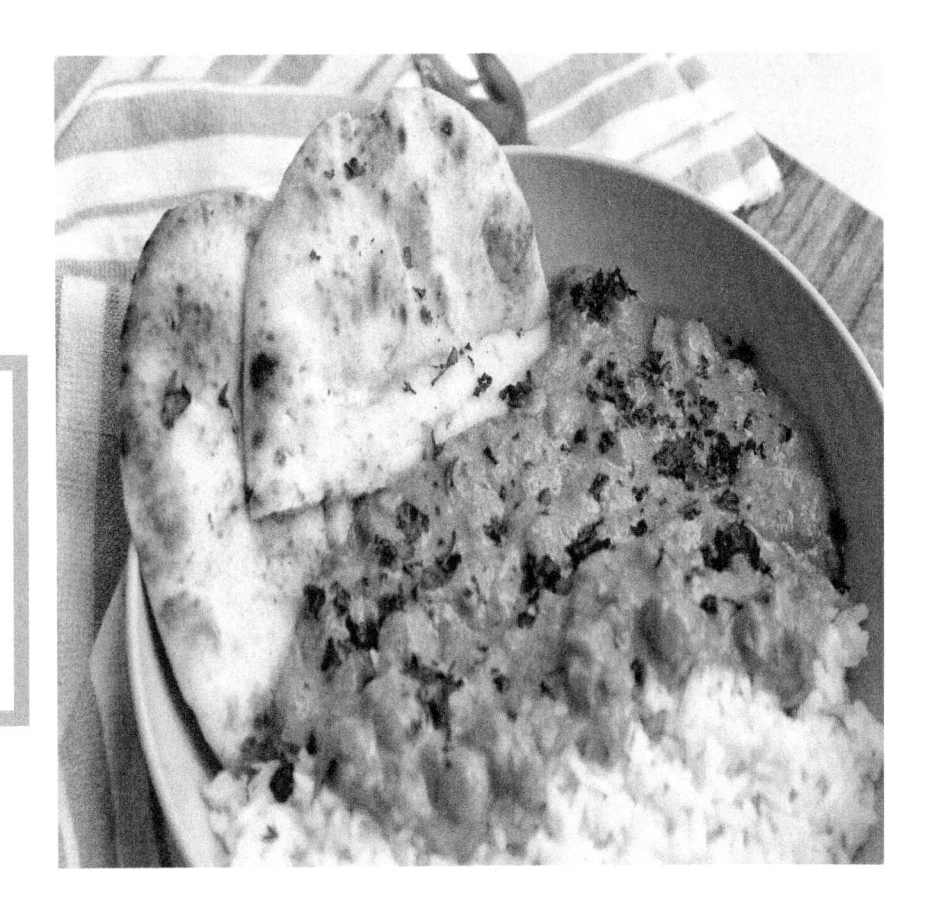

Ingredients

Salt to taste	1 tsp ground coriander
1/2 tsp ground turmeric	1 1/8 cups diced tomatoes with juice
1 can chickpeas	6 tsp ground turmeric
1-inch piece of fresh ginger	1/2 medium chopped yellow onion
2 large garlic cloves	1 tsp ground cumin
3 tbsp canola oil	

Instructions

1. Using a food processor, mince the serrano chiles, garlic, and onion until the ingredients are uniformly dispersed throughout the mixture. When scraping the sides of the blender, give the mixture one more twirl in the blender. Once you've added the onion, please give it a few pulses in the stick blender until it's broken down into small pieces but isn't completely liquidized.

2. Place the oil in a large saucepan and heat it over medium-high heat until it reaches a simmering temperature. After adding the onion combination, continue cooking it for five minutes while giving this a toss now and then until it becomes softer. The cooking procedure should be maintained for another two minutes while stirring after adding the mustard, ginger, and turmeric.

3. The tomatoes should be crushed in spice crushers until they reach a consistency similar to a very fine powder. In this process step, you should also add salt to the current ingredients in the pan. Cook the mixture for four minutes at a simmer, during which time you should stir it often and maintain the temperature at the same level. After adding the chickpeas and the curry powder, reduce the heat to a medium-low setting and maintain that setting throughout the cooking process. Cook the food for another five minutes with the lid on, stirring or flipping the contents of the pot at regular intervals. You may give it with a little chopped cilantro if you think it would be helpful.

| **Nutrition Facts** | Calories: 300 calories, Proteins: 3.9 g, Carbs: 9 g, Fat: 2.8 g |

7.7: Mushroom Sauce Meatloaf

Prep Time: 35 minutes

Cook Time: 1 hour

Servings: 1

Difficulty level: Difficult

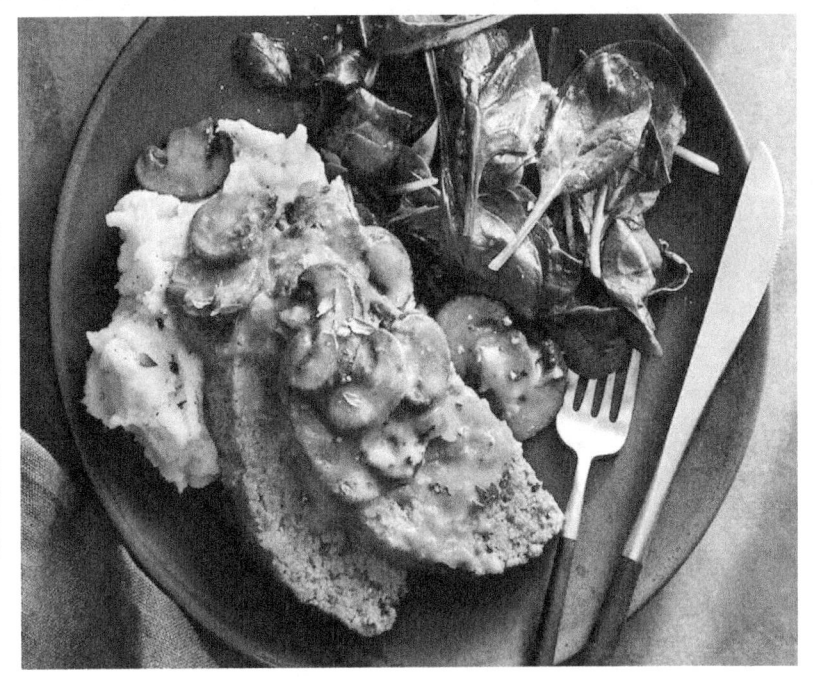

Ingredients

Egg white 1	Sour cream 100 g
Garlic clove 0.5	Breadcrumbs 3/4 cup
Salt 1/8 tsp	Milk 2 tbsp
Butter 0.5 tbsp	Pepper 1/16 tsp
Flour 1 tbsp	Cold water 3/8 cup
Mushrooms 3/4 cup	Green onions 2 tbsp
Beef 0.225 kg	Bouillon beef 1 tsp
Italian seasoning 1 tsp	

Instructions

1. Set the temperature of the ovens to 176 degrees Centigrade (350 degrees Fahrenheit). Place aside a rectangular baking dish that has been covered in aluminum foil and has a capacity of two quarts.
2. Using a fork, thoroughly combine the egg whites and milk in a dish until no streaks of either ingredient are left.
3. The mixture is then given chopped spring onions, crumbs, a quarter cup of sliced salt, Italian

seasoning, and an eighth of a teaspoon of pepper.

4. Ensure that the ground beef is mixed up completely before proceeding. In the dish, you will be baking, shape the meat mixture into a rectangle 7 inches in diameter and 4 inches tall.
5. Place the dish in the oven and bake for about 1 hour and 45 minutes, or till a core temperature measurement of 71.1 degrees Centigrade (160 ° Fahrenheit) is attained.
6. Position the thermometer to read the beef loaf's internal temperature and determine whether it has been cooked.
7. Using a spoon, scrape out any excess fat from the pan. Before cutting into the meatloaf and serving it, let it rest for 10 minutes.
8. Move the meatloaf to the serving tray using two spatulas and drain any extra fat.
9. Meanwhile, prepare the sauce by coating a medium-sized skillet with cooking spray. To get started, place the butter in a saucepan of medium size and bring it up to a simmer over medium heat.
10. After about four minutes of cooking, while constantly turning the pan, ensure the mushrooms are almost entirely cooked.
11. After adding a quart container of chopped green onions, continue to cook for one additional minute after adding the green onions. In a basin designated for that purpose, cream and wheat should be combined.
12. Combine the chopped mushrooms, chicken bouillon cubes, and cold water in a large bowl. Blend until smooth.
13. In a saucepan, stir together the mushroom and crème combinations until the ingredients are well combined. Keep heating the sauce while stirring it often until it reaches the required consistency and begins to bubble.
14. Toss the ingredients and continue to heat them for one further minute. To attain the desired level of thinness, it may be necessary to add more water; do so if necessary.
15. When the meatloaf is served, the sauce should be drizzled on top of it. It is recommended that more pepper plus chopped green onions be sprinkled over the top, although this is optional.

Nutrition Facts	Calories: 214 calories, Proteins: 21 g, Carbs: 9 g, Fat: 9g.

7.8: Pressure Cooker Apple Chicken

Prep Time: 25 minutes

Cook Time: 20 minutes

Servings: 1

Difficulty level: Easy

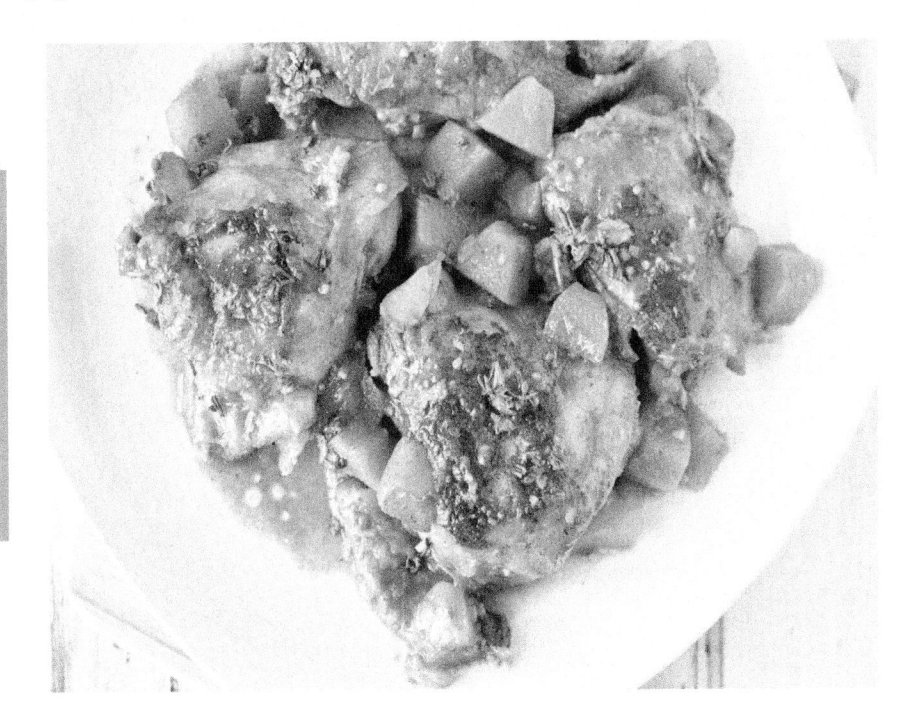

Ingredients

1/4 teaspoon salt	1/3 cup barbecue sauce
1 garlic clove	1 medium onion, sliced
1/4 teaspoon pepper	1/2 cup apple cider
1 chicken thigh	1 tablespoon oil
1 tablespoon honey	

Instructions

1. Sprinkle the chicken with salt and pepper when it has been prepared. Browning or sautéing may be done in a pressure cooker with a capacity of six quarts using the appropriate setting.

2. The temperature must be reduced to medium, and oil should be added. After the oil has been heated, brown the chicken, take it from the pan and keep it warm.

3. Once you've added the cider and mixed it, scrape the browned bits from the bottom of the

bread pan. Before adding the chicken, combine the onion, honey, bbq sauce, and garlic in a mixing bowl.

4. Ensure the safety valve is closed and the lid is locked before proceeding. Make the appropriate modifications to cooking the food for 10 minutes under high pressure.

5. After letting the pressure subside for five minutes, rapidly alleviate any pressure that may still be there.

6. A thermometer inside the bird should register at least 170 degrees Centigrade before being removed.

7. Take the chicken out of the pan and keep it warm.

8. Using the menu, choose the sauté function and lower the temperature to a low setting.

9. Once you have added the apples, cook the mixture while mixing it for around 10 minutes until they become tender.

10. Complete the preparation with chicken and then serve.

| **Nutrition Facts** | Calories: 340 calories, Proteins: 25 g, Carbs: 31 g, Fat: 13 g. |

7.9: Baked Salmon with Roasted Broccoli

Prep Time: 15 minutes

Cook Time: 10 minutes

Servings: 1

Difficulty level: Easy

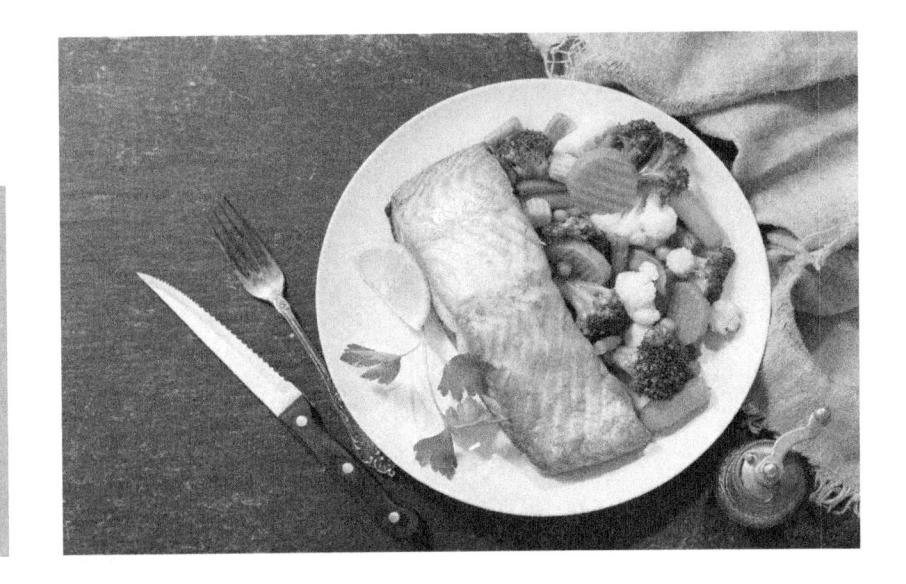

Ingredients

4 salmon fillets	1 lemon, sliced
1 tbsp. olive oil	2 cloves of garlic, minced
Salt and pepper, to taste	1 large head of florets broccoli

Instructions

1. Turn the oven up to 0400 degrees Fahrenheit.
2. A baking sheet should be prepared with parchment paper.
3. Arrange the salmon skins/fillets in a single layer on the baking sheet that has been prepared.
4. Salt and pepper the fish, drizzle it with olive oil and season it with salt.
5. Cook the salmon in the oven for 12 to 15 minutes or until it reaches the desired doneness.
6. Toss the broccoli florets with minced garlic, freshly ground black pepper, & kosher salt in a large basin.
7. Put together the broccoli in a single layer on a separate baking sheet, and roast it in the oven for 012 to 015 minutes, until it is fork-tender and has a light golden brown color.
8. Salmon that has been baked should be served with roasted broccoli and sliced lemons.

Nutrition Facts Calories: 360 calories, Proteins: 34g, Carbs: 10g, Fat: 20g

7.10: Turkey Chili

Prep Time: 15 minutes

Cook Time: 10 minutes

Servings: 1

Difficulty level: Easy

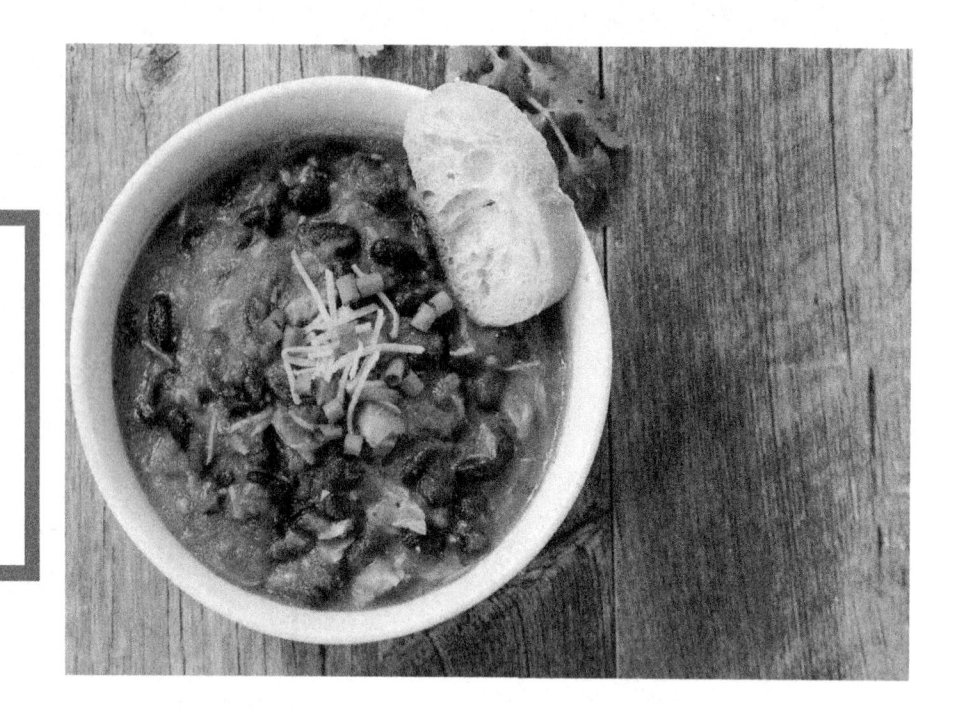

Ingredients

1 lb. ground turkey	1 tsp. dried oregano
Salt and pepper	1 tsp. ground cumin
1 tbsp. olive oil	1 tbsp. chili powder
1 large onion, chopped	1 can of kidney beans, drained & rinsed
2 cloves of garlic, minced	1 can of chopped tomatoes

Instructions

1. In a large pot, cook/heat the olive oil around medium heat.
2. Add the chopped onion & minced garlic and cook until the onion is soft & translucent.
3. Add the ground turkey and cook until browned and fully cooked.
4. Stir in the diced tomatoes, kidney beans, chili powder, cumin, oregano, salt, and pepper.
5. Reduce heat and simmer for 20-25 minutes until the flavors have melded together.
6. Serve the turkey chili hot, and enjoy!

Nutrition Facts Calories: 328 calories, Proteins: 28g, Carbs: 27g, Fat: 13g

Chapter 8: Soups and Stews Recipes

8.1: Tummy Healing Soup

Prep Time: 30 minutes

Cook Time: 50 minutes

Servings: 1

Difficulty level: Easy

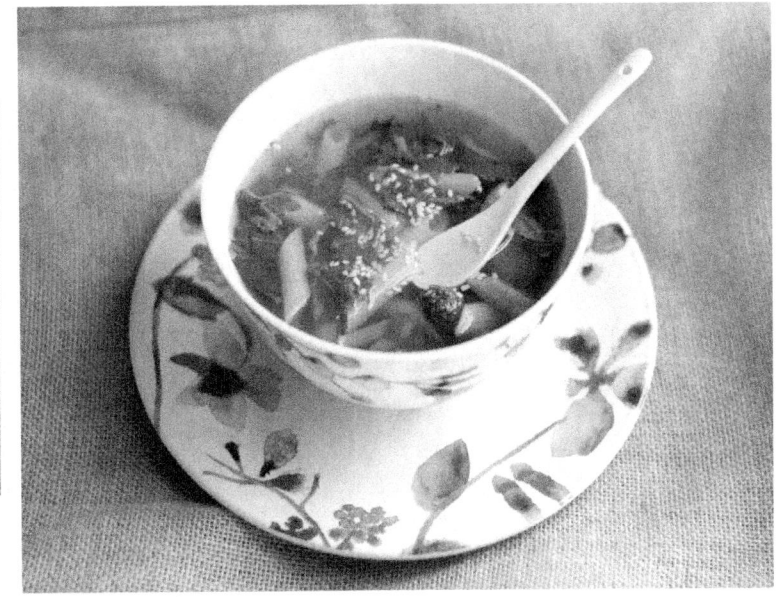

Ingredients

1/4 tsp minced garlic	1 tsp coconut aminos
3/4 cup water	1/4 tsp Chinese 5 spice
1/4 cup gluten-free penne	1/4 cup chopped broccoli rabe
1/4 tsp toasted sesame seeds	1/4 tsp ground ginger
1-inch piece of turmeric root	2 tbsp dried porcini mushrooms

Instructions

1. Place the garlic, ginger, turmeric, and five spice in a small pot with three cups of water. Stir to combine. On the burner, bring to a rolling boil.
2. Now stir in the broccoli rabe, mushrooms, and penne pasta until everything is well combined. Turn the heat up down to moderate and cook for another 5 minutes.
3. After adding the coconut aminos, transfer the mixture to a large soup dish. If you'd like, sprinkle some sesame seeds on top.

Nutrition Facts   Calories: 320 calories, Proteins: 23g, Carbs: 34g, Fat: 4g

8.2: Onion Thyme Soup

Prep Time: 30 minutes

Cook Time: 30 minutes

Servings: 1

Difficulty level: Easy

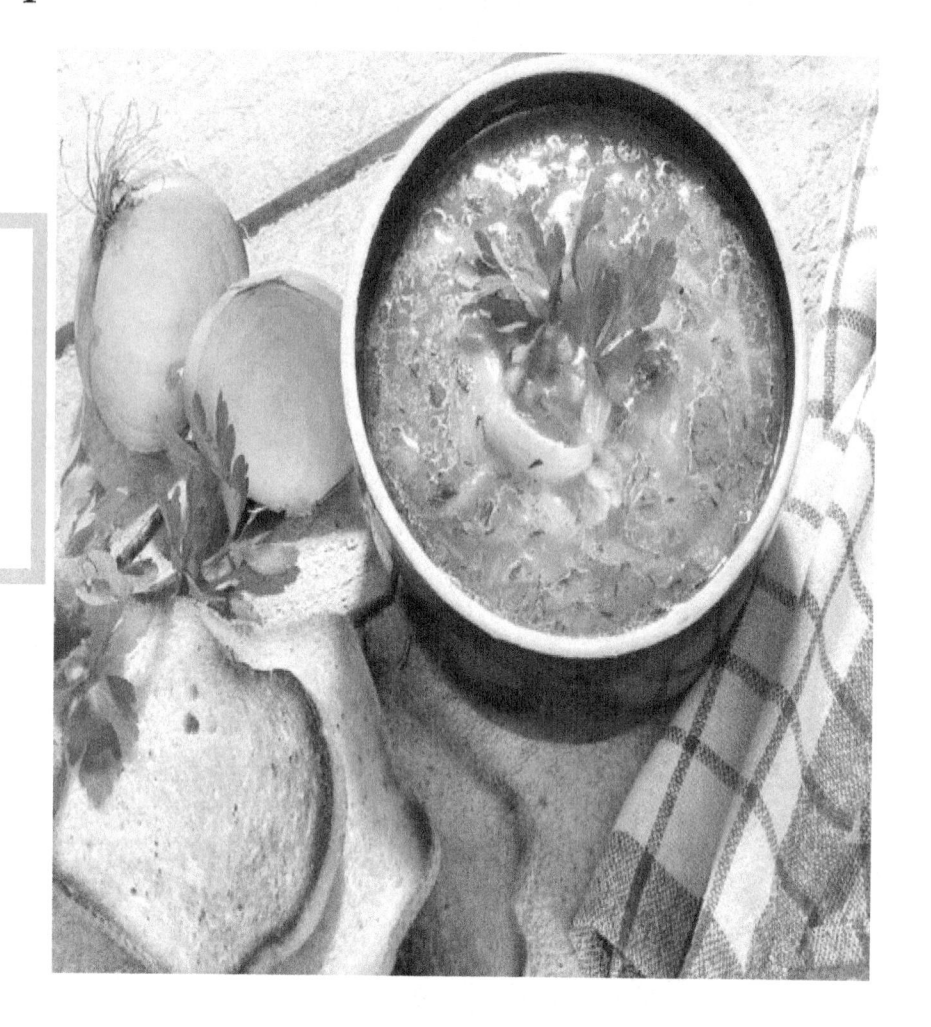

Ingredients

1/8 cup celery, chopped	1 sprig of coriander leaves
1/4 cup chopped spring onions	2 teaspoons low-fat butter
1/4 cup chopped carrots	1 tablespoon thyme
1 cup water	1 teaspoon black pepper
1 tablespoon whole wheat flour	Black pepper and salt to taste

Instructions

1. Prepare the vegetables by dicing them and then boiling them.

2. Put eight cups of water into a pan with a deep bottom and non-stick coating, then add chopped carrots, one cup of chopped onions, minced celery, sprigs of coriander, and ground black pepper. Bring the mixture to a boil. While swirling the mixture occasionally, thoroughly combine the components.

3. Sauté the vegetables over low heat, then drain the stock.

4. Cook the meat over low heat for twenty minutes while the cover is on the pan. Do not forget to whisk the ingredients together at regular intervals.

5. After everything is finished, strain any vegetable stock through a sieve. Throw away all veggies, but put the stock in a separate container for later use.

6. Heat butter and sauté vegetables

7. Warm the butter in a skillet with a deep bottom that does not stick and set it aside. After the melted butter, add the onions to the pan and roast them over standard heat for a few minutes or until brown.

8. Next, add chopped scallions, thyme, and whole wheat flour to the pan. Mix everything thoroughly, then sauté the mixture for several seconds over a medium temperature.

9. Cook the mixture after adding the vegetable stock.

10. When the mixture is finished cooking, combine everything thoroughly in the vegetable stock. To keep the dish's flavor and aroma, season it to taste with salt and pepper and thoroughly combine the ingredients.

11. Remember to stir the mixture occasionally while cooking over a medium-intensity burner for a few minutes. The Onions Thyme Soup is finished when garnished with coriander sprigs and ready to be consumed immediately.

Nutrition Facts   Calories: 200 calories, Proteins: 24g, Carbs: 23g, Fat: 3g

8.3: Broccoli and Sweet Potato Soup

Prep Time: 20 minutes

Cook Time: 40 minutes

Servings: 1

Difficulty level: Easy

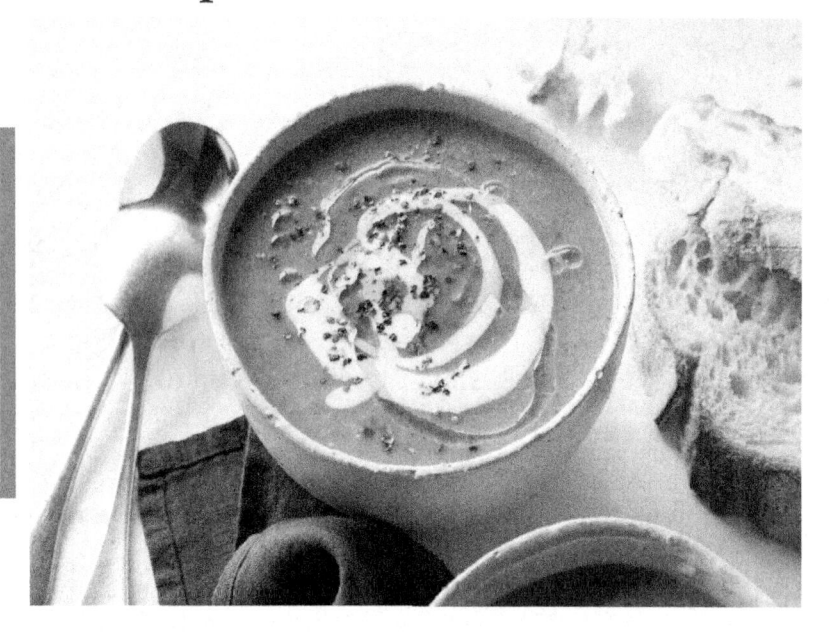

Ingredients

1 medium onion	1/4 medium broccoli head
1 medium sweet potato	1 tsp light olive oil
1 small garlic clove	1 tsp vegetable stock
1 small handful of kale	

Instructions

1. The oil should be heated in a huge pan or wok over low heat.

2. After the oil has been heated, add the minced onion and garlic, and cook over low heat for about 4-5 minutes. Watch out that the onions don't get too charred. Mix it up every so often.

3. When the sweet potatoes have been chopped, add them to the pan or wok and mix them thoroughly. To give it a little extra spice, sprinkle in specific stock Spicy.

4. Cover the saucepan and set aside for approximately three to four minutes while you prepare the vegetable stock.

5. Once the stock is finished, pour it onto the pan and whisk everything together until it is completely incorporated.

6. After bringing the potatoes to a boil with the lid on, decrease the warmth and let them simmer for 5 min.

7. After washing and chopping the kale and broccoli, add them to the pan. Ensure all ingredients are submerged in the liquid; add more water.

8. Bring the tap water back up to a cook, cut the heat to low and continue to simmer for another 8-10 minutes with the lid on the pan. Make sure to stir the mixture occasionally.

9. After it has been taken to a simmer, transfer the soup ingredients into a food processor or blender and process it until it is completely smooth and creamy.

10. Mix in some sprouts, and then sprinkle some stock on top.

| **Nutrition Facts** | Calories: 230 calories, Proteins: 34g, Carbs: 21g, Fat: 2g |

8.4: Cabbage Stew

Prep Time: 30 minutes

Cook Time: 50 minutes

Servings: 1

Difficulty level: Easy

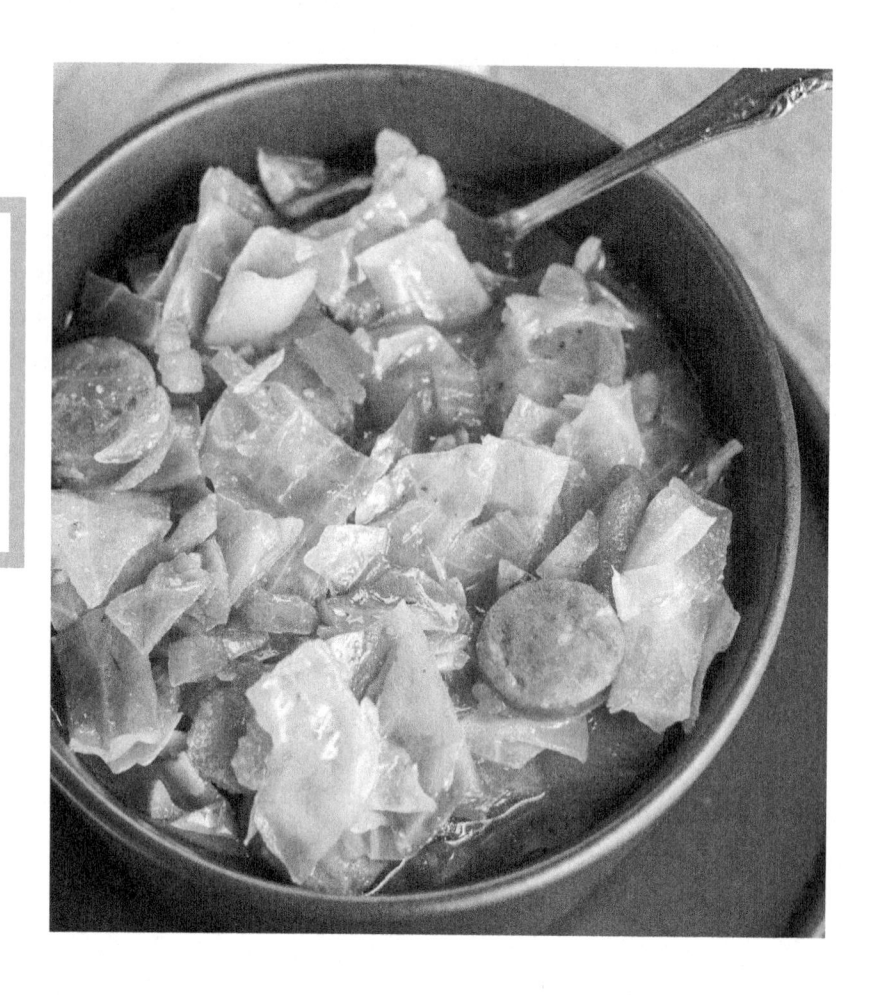

Ingredients

1 tsp Salt	1/2 tsp Pepper
1/8 cup diced tomatoes	1/2 tsp Ginger
1/2 tsp Garlic	2 tbsp Carrots chopped
1/2 tsp Dried Oregano	1/4 cup Celery diced
2 tbsp Capsicum diced	3 cups Vegetable Stock
1/2 tsp Red Chilli flakes	4-5 Fresh Basil leaves roughly torn
1/4 cup chopped onion	3/4 cup chopped cabbage
1 1/2 tbsp Olive oil	Parsley chopped

Instructions

1. Ginger and garlic should be fried for about half a minute after being added to oil heated in a big saucepan — Fry for a further half a minute after adding the onions. After adding the celery, carrots, cabbage, and Capsicum, simmer the mixture for another three to four minutes.

2. After adding the tomatoes, salt, and stock, bring the mix to a boil and then reduce the heat to a simmer for around twenty minutes.

3. Add the herbs, pepper, and chili flakes to the dish. Combine thoroughly. To serve, bring to a boil and top with chopped fresh parsley.

4. Sauté the food in the instant pot by selecting the sauté function and heating the oil. Fry the ginger and garlic for half a minute after adding them. Fry for a further half a minute after adding the onions. After adding the salt and stock, stir in the celery, onions, cabbage, Capsicum, and tomatoes. Ensure the lid is securely fastened, then switch the valve to the sealing mode. The high pressure should be set for two minutes. After allowing the pressure to drop naturally for ten minutes, the pressure should then be released manually.

5. Mix in the dried herbs, red pepper flakes, and black pepper. To serve, bring to a boil and top with chopped fresh parsley.

6. The consumption of cabbage can assist in the elimination of toxins and extra fluid from the body due to its diuretic characteristics. It aids in the cleansing of both your liver and intestines. This detoxifying cabbage soup relies heavily on the cabbage as its foundational ingredient for a good reason.

7. You can include vegetables or protein, such as eggs, ground chicken, or lamb!

8. Keep in the refrigerator for up to a week when stored in an airtight container. Reheat the food every time before serving.

Nutrition Facts   Calories: 330 calories, Proteins: 24g, Carbs: 24g, Fat: 3g

8.5: Chicken Soup Stew

Prep Time: 30 minutes

Cook Time: 50 minutes

Servings: 1

Difficulty level: Easy

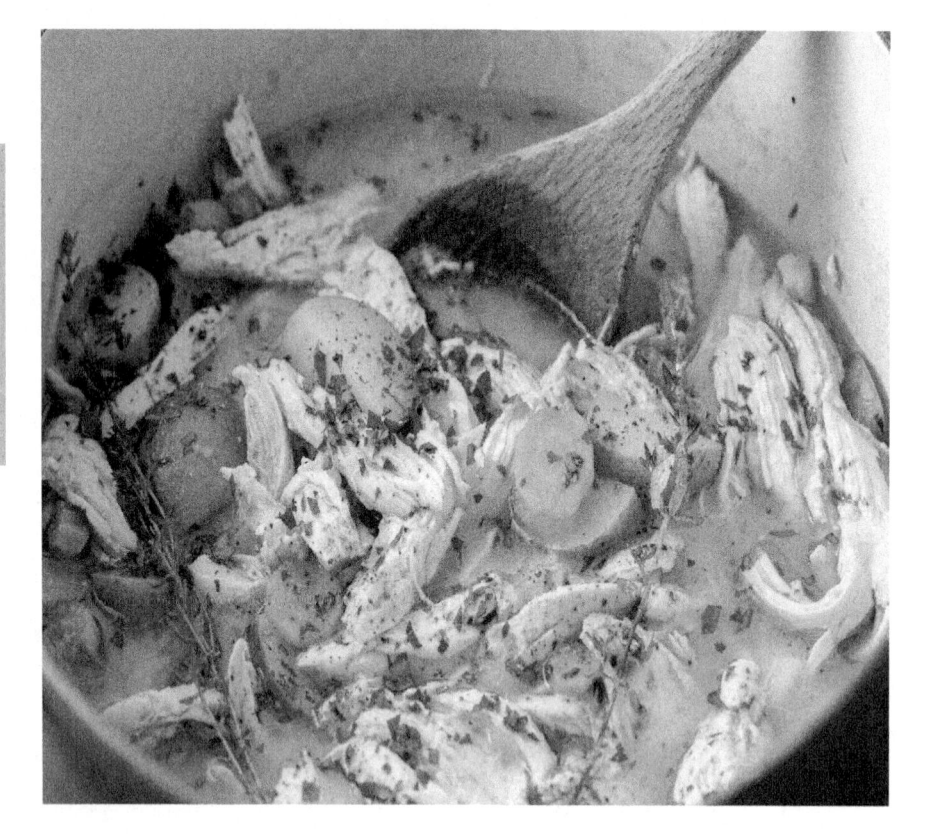

Ingredients

1 tbsp Butter	1 Whole Clove
250g Chicken	1 tsp Lemon Juice
1 tbsp Refined Vegetable Oil	1 small Tomato
1 Cinnamon Stick	1 tsp Turmeric Powder
4-5 French Bean	5 Whole Black Pepper
1 tsp Crushed Black Pepper	1/2 Raw Papaya
1 tsp Bengali Garam Masala Powder	Salt to taste
1 tsp Garlic Paste	1/2 Onion
1 tsp Ginger Paste	1/2 Carrot
1 Potato	

Instructions

1. After thoroughly cleaning the chicken pieces, marinate them in lemon juice, turmeric powder, and a half teaspoon of salt.

2. Potato, carrot, tomato, and raw papaya should be sliced into long strips (as seen in the picture), and the onion should be cut into large chunks.

3. Now, take a crock pot and make sure that 1 tablespoon of purified vegetable oil is heated to the correct temperature. While the oil is still hot, season it with all of the spices.

4. Sauté the chopped onions and ginger-garlic paste for one minute after adding them to the pan.

5. Add the Marinated Chicken Pieces and the vegetables to the tempering, and mix everything nicely with a spatula.

6. Mix in some pepper powder and salt according to your preferences, then add the salt to the chicken & mix it up.

7. Now, continue stirring while you cook for another two to three minutes.

8. To the mixture, add the necessary amount of water. The chicken-veggie combination must be covered entirely in water.

9. After placing the Pressure Canner weight inside, cover it cooker with the lid, and then begin cooking over a medium temperature. Continue cooking until the cooker makes three whistles.

10. Please turn off the flame and lift the cover when the pressure has returned to its original level. At this point, you could smell the fantastic Bengali Chicken Stew.

11. Afterward, include the Curry Paste Powder and the Butter in the Stew. Adding butter is entirely discretionary but will undoubtedly enhance Stew's flavor.

| **Nutrition Facts** | Calories: 330 calories, Proteins: 45g, Carbs: 10g, Fat: 2g |

8.6: Harvest Soup

Prep Time: 10 minutes

Cook Time: 20 minutes

Servings: 1

Difficulty level: Medium

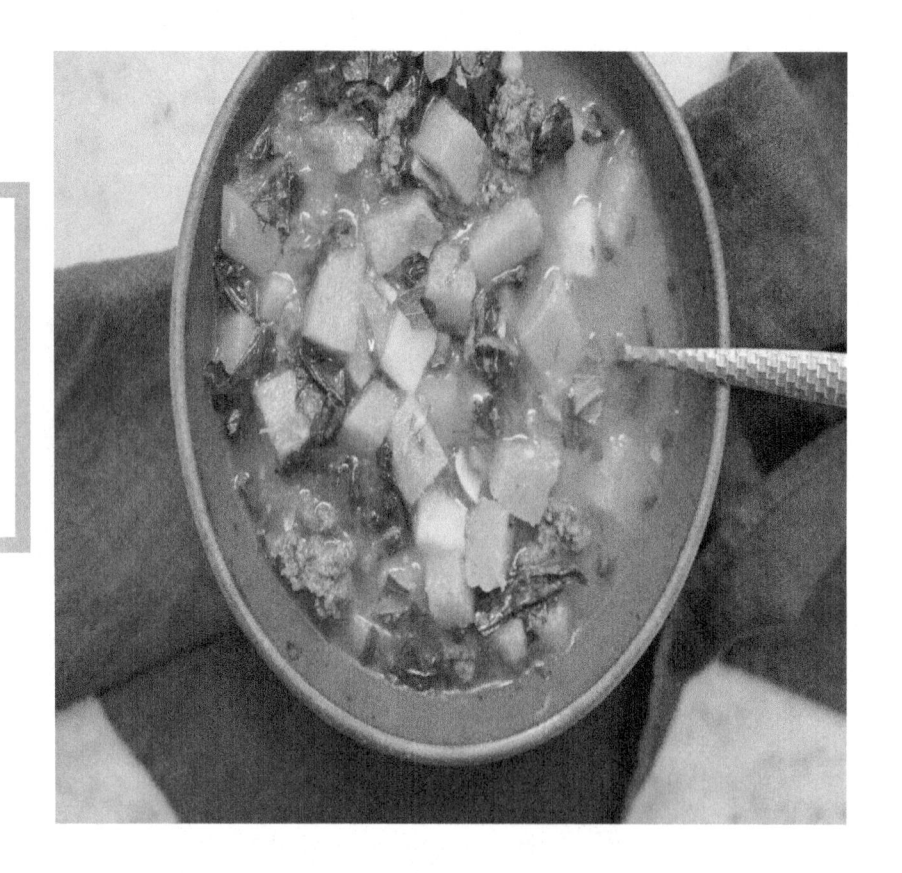

Ingredients

2 tablespoons cream of chicken soup	1 turkey breast
Chicken stock	1 teaspoon seasoning

Instructions

1. Turkey should be processed in a blender until it is powdered.
2. Blend in the soup and season until smooth.
3. Add chicken broth until the soup has the consistency you want.

Nutrition Facts   Calories: 200 calories, Proteins: 12g, Carbs: 23g, Fat: 9g

8.7: Spicy Bean Soup

Prep Time: 20 minutes

Cook Time: 30 minutes

Servings: 1

Difficulty level: Medium

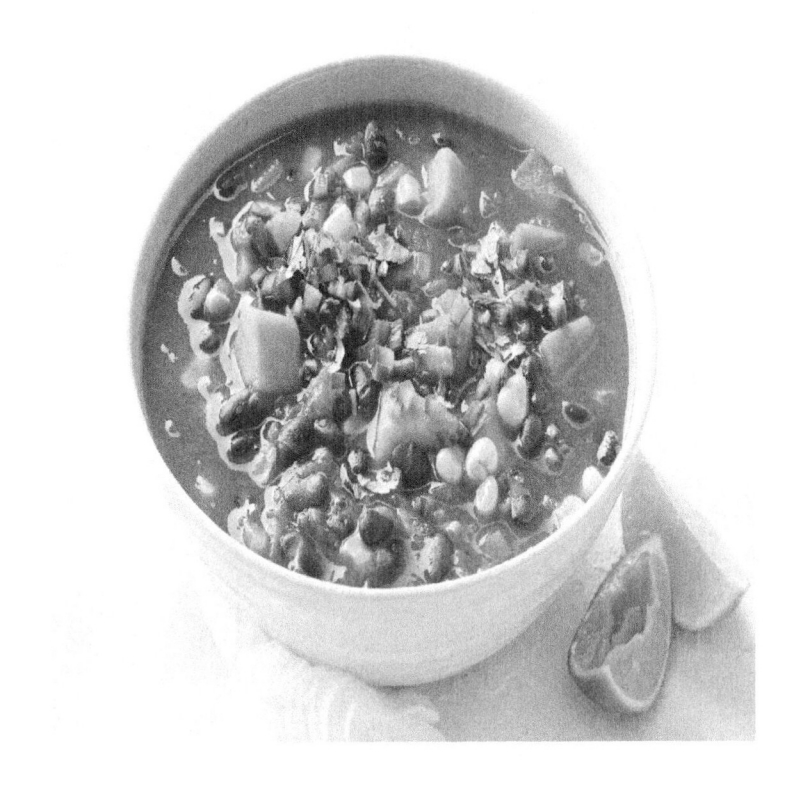

Ingredients

1 cup of refried beans	½ cup salsa
6 deli chicken	8 fat-free milk

Instructions

1. Chicken should be coarsely ground after being placed in a food processor and pulsed.

2. Refried beans should be added and blended further until smooth.

3. Blend until smooth while adding evaporated skim milk or nonfat milk. If necessary, chicken broth can be added to thicken the soup.

4. Until you are ready to use, please place it in the refrigerator.

Nutrition Facts Calories: 230 calories, Proteins: 14g, Carbs: 31g, Fat: 12g

8.8: Healing Vegetable Soup

Prep Time: 10 minutes

Cook Time: 30 minutes

Servings: 1

Difficulty level: Easy

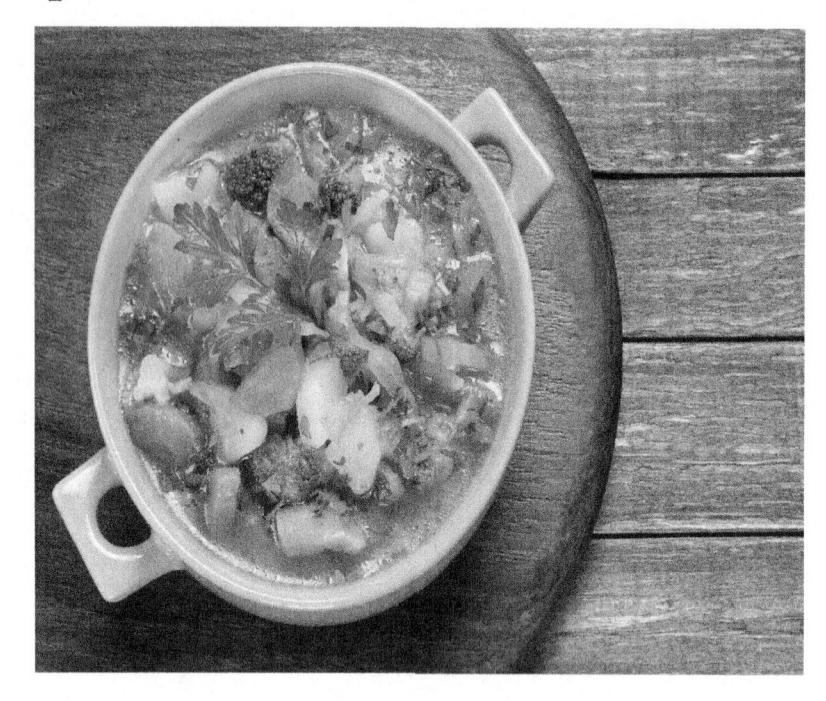

Ingredients

Low-sodium vegetable broth	1 small zucchini, diced
1 small yellow squash, diced	1 small carrot, diced
1 small onion, diced	1 small garlic clove, minced
1/2 tsp dried thyme	1/4 tsp black pepper

Instructions

1. In a medium saucepan, heat the vegetable broth over medium heat.
2. Add diced zucchini, carrot, yellow squash, onion, garlic, dried thyme, and black pepper to the broth.
3. Cook for 25-30 minutes until the vegetables are tender.
4. Then, blend the ingredients until they reach a smooth texture and serve the soup hot.

Nutrition Facts   Calories: 120 calories, Proteins: 4g, Carbs: 25g, Fat: 2g

8.9: Veggie Lentil Soup

Prep Time: 15 minutes

Cook Time: 45 minutes

Servings: 1

Difficulty level: Easy

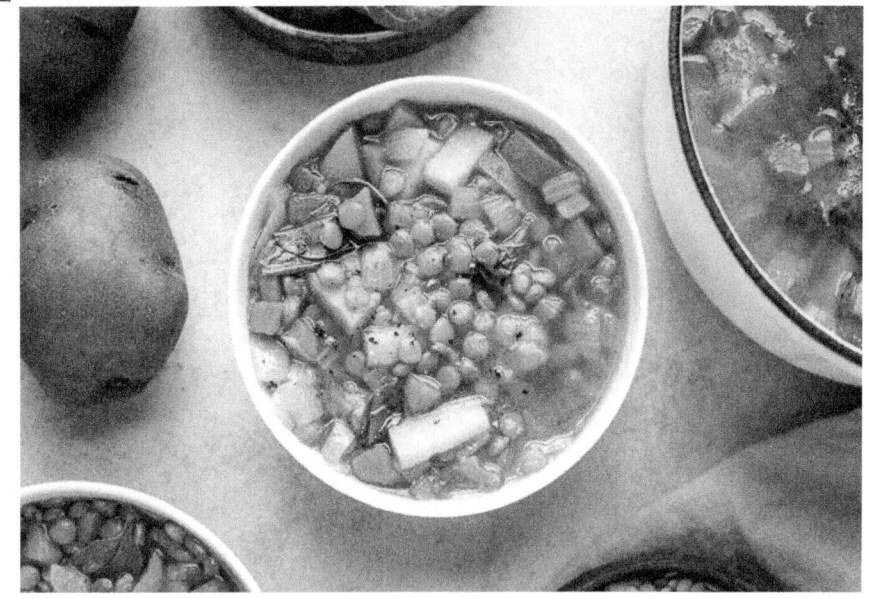

Ingredients

1/4 cup green or brown lentils	Salt and pepper, to taste
1 large carrot, diced	1/4 tsp dried rosemary
1 celery stalk, diced	1/4 tsp dried thyme
1/4 onion, diced	3 cups low-sodium vegetable broth
1 garlic clove, minced	1 tbsp olive oil

Instructions

1. Rinse the lentils and keep them aside.
2. In a pot, heat the olive oil over medium heat.
3. Once heated, add diced carrots, celery, onion, and garlic and cook until the vegetables are soft and translucent, around 5 minutes.
4. Mix in dried thyme and rosemary, followed by the lentils.
5. Pour the vegetable broth into the pot and bring the mixture to a boil.
6. Lower the heat and let the soup simmer until the lentils are tender, for about 30-35 minutes.
7. Taste and season with salt and pepper as desired.
8. Enjoy the soup hot.

Nutrition Facts Calories: 250 calories, Proteins: 12g, Carbs: 40g, Fat: 7g

8.10: Grilled Chicken Broth Bowl

Prep Time: 15 minutes

Cook Time: 30 minutes

Servings: 1

Difficulty level: Easy

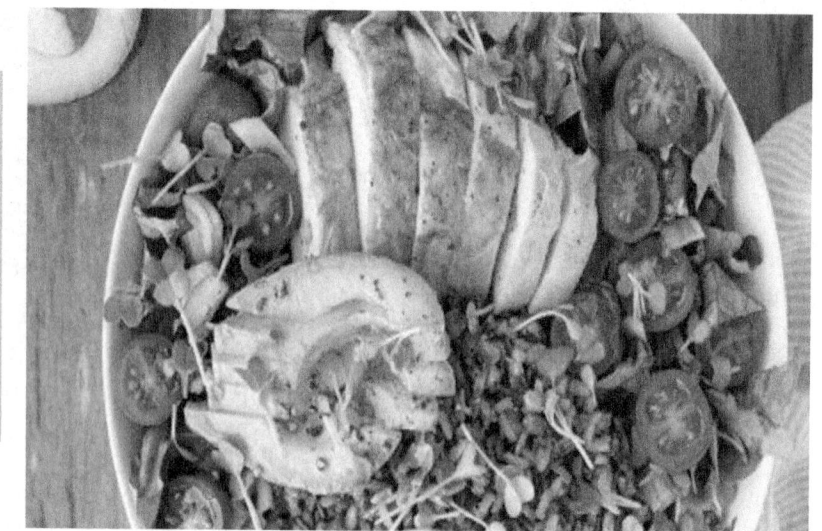

Ingredients

1 cup low-sodium chicken broth	1 garlic clove, minced
1 boneless, skinless chicken breast	1 teaspoon dried thyme
1/2 cup chopped carrots	1 teaspoon dried rosemary
1/2 cup chopped zucchini	1 teaspoon olive oil
1/2 cup chopped bell peppers	Salt and pepper to taste

Instructions

1. Warm the chicken broth in a small saucepan over medium heat. Keep it warm until ready to use.
2. Heat olive oil over medium-high heat in a separate pan and sauté garlic, carrots, zucchini, and bell peppers until tender, approximately 5-7 minutes.
3. Season chicken breast with thyme, rosemary, salt, and pepper and add to the pan. Cook until the chicken is fully cooked and reaches an internal temperature of 165°F, around 8-10 minutes per side.
4. Once the chicken is cooked, cut it into bite-sized pieces and divide it among bowls with the sautéed vegetables.
5. Serve by pouring the warm chicken broth over the top. Enjoy immediately.

Nutrition Facts Calories: 250 calories, Protein: 26g, Carbs: 20g, Fat: 8g

Chapter 9: Puree Recipes

9.1: Sweet Salmon Puree

Prep Time: 15 minutes

Cook Time: 30 minutes

Servings: 1

Difficulty level: Medium

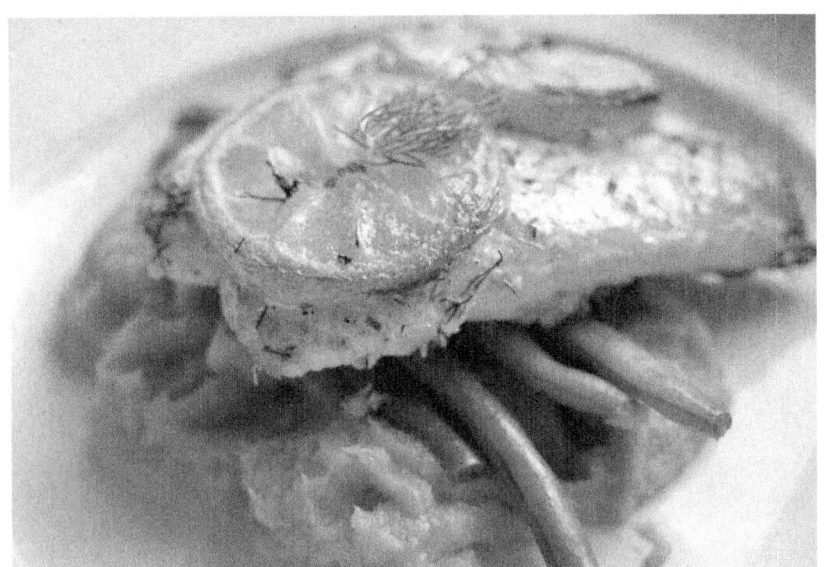

Ingredients

Vegetable stock	Frozen peas
1 large sweet potato	2 salmon

Instructions

1. Add the stock to a big saucepan and cook it over medium heat. Then add other vegetables after bringing them to a boil.
2. Simmer for 15 minutes. Add the fish to the skillet after the sweet potatoes start to soften.
3. For around 8 to 10 minutes, cover and poach the fish. Please ensure there are no little bones in the salmon before removing it and flaking it into a big basin. Blend the vegetables after placing them in a blender.
4. Place the fish on vegetables in your pots. If you are unfamiliar with texture, you might also puree the salmon.
5. Extra parts should be frozen for later use.

Nutrition Facts — Calories: 230 calories, Proteins: 10g, Carbs: 45g, Fat: 8g

9.2: Avocado Puree

Prep Time: 5 minutes

Cook Time: 0 minutes

Servings: 1

Difficulty level: Medium

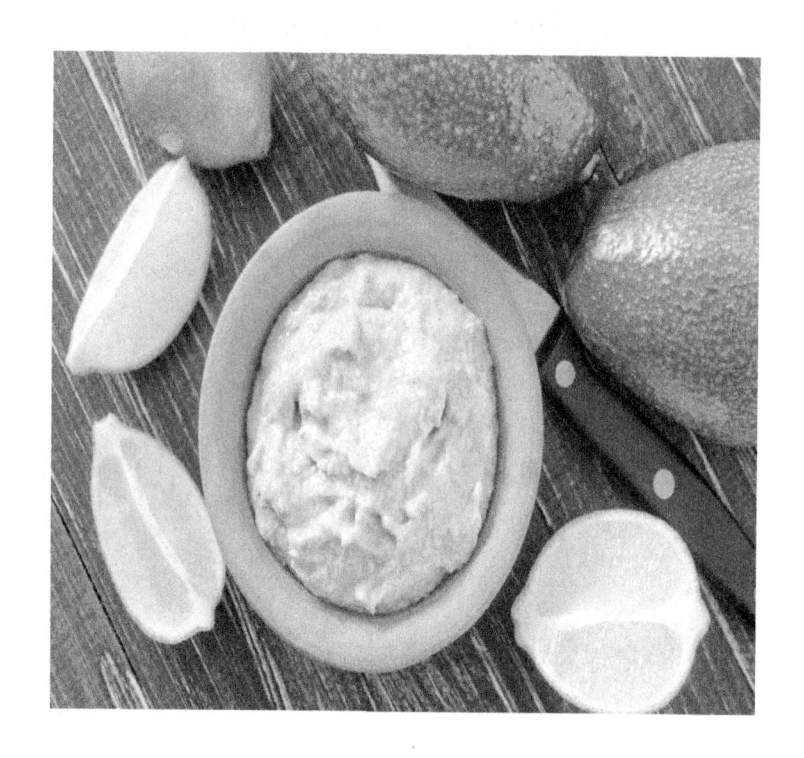

Ingredients

Vegetable stock	Frozen peas
1 large sweet potato	2 salmon

Instructions

1. Slice the avocado in half. After that, remove the flesh. You'll have at least 1 cup to make this in a blender.

2. Include in a blender. I am starting on low, mixing until smooth, thinning as necessary with a bit of water, milk, or formula to achieve the desired smoothness.

3. Serve right away.

4. Place purée into little food plastic tubs and cover with freshly squeezed lemon juice to keep. Remove any exposed areas with lemon juice to stop the puree from browning.

Nutrition Facts	Calories: 150 calories, Proteins: 50g, Carbs: 15g, Fat: 5g

9.3: Mango and Peanut Butter Puree

Prep Time: 5 minutes

Cook Time: 5 minutes

Servings: 1

Difficulty level: Medium

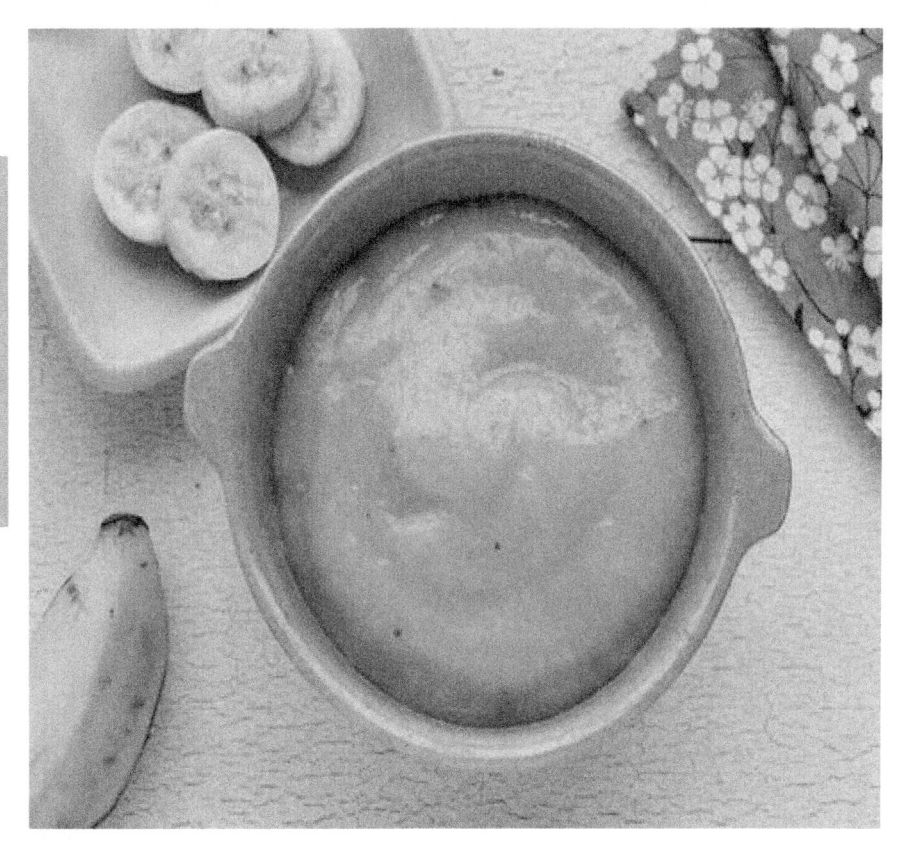

Ingredients

2 bananas	¼ cup coconut milk
2 Tablespoon peanut butter	1 cup mango

Instructions

1. Mango, banana, and peanut butter should all be thoroughly blended.

2. Add coconut milk or baby's regular milk until the texture is as desired.

Nutrition Facts   Calories: 250 calories, Proteins: 15g, Carbs: 23g, Fat: 12g

9.4: Vegetable Soup Puree

Prep Time: 5 minutes

Cook Time: 5 minutes

Servings: 1

Difficulty level: Medium

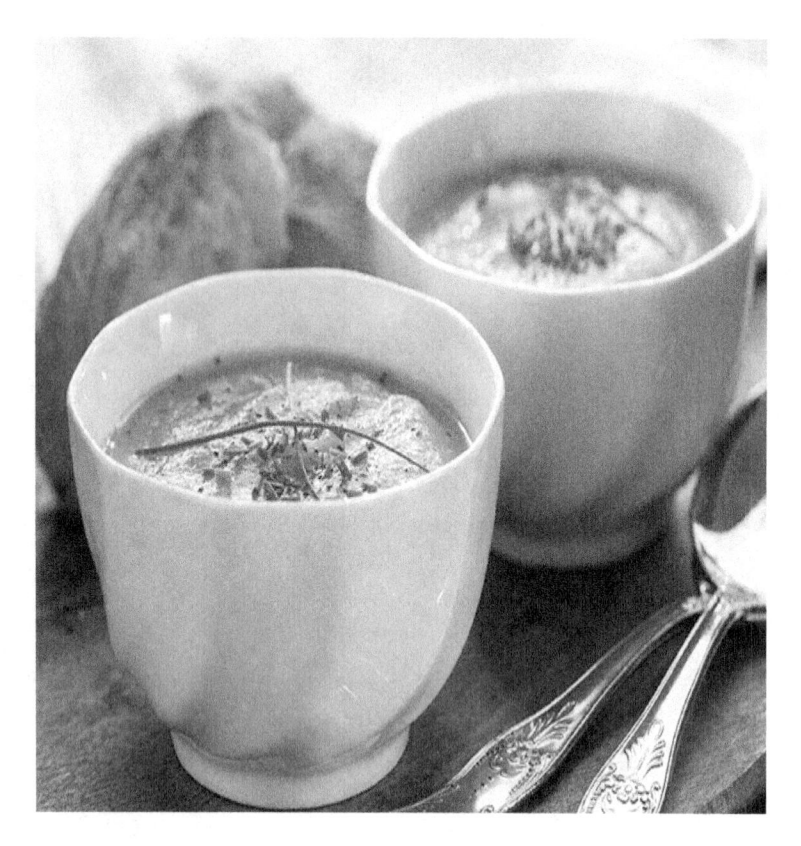

Ingredients

Black pepper	Vegetables
Vegetable broth	Salt

Instructions

1. Assemble the components.

2. The vegetables & broth should be combined in a big pot. All veggies should be soft before simmering partially covered at low heat. Please bring it to a boil over high heat.

3. Salt and pepper the soup, then purée it with an immersion blender until smooth.

Nutrition Facts   Calories: 150 calories, Proteins: 25g, Carbs:12g, Fat:6g

9.5: Pumpkin Puree

Prep Time: 25 minutes

Cook Time: 30 minutes

Servings: 1

Difficulty level: Medium

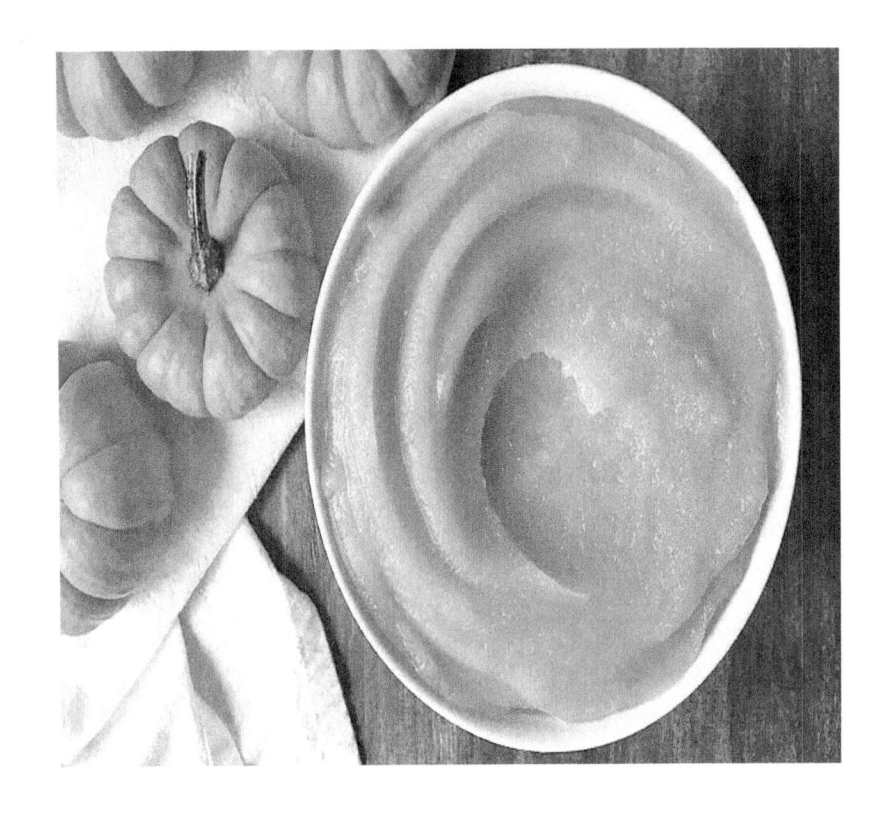

Ingredients

Paprika	Pumpkin
Chicken broth	Sugar
Olive oil	Curry powder
1 clove garlic	Medium onion

Instructions

1. Oil is cooked over medium-high heat in a 3-quart pan. When the onion is crisp-tender, add the onion and garlic and simmer for 1 to 2 minutes, turning constantly.
2. Add the remaining ingredients and stir. Reduce heat to low, and boil for 10 to 12 minutes or until veggies are soft, stirring occasionally. Add pepper, if required, to taste.

Nutrition Facts Calories: 250 calories, Proteins: 12g, Carbs: 23g, Fat: 10g

9.6: Mix Vegetable Puree

Prep Time: 25 minutes

Cook Time: 30 minutes

Servings: 1

Difficulty level: Medium

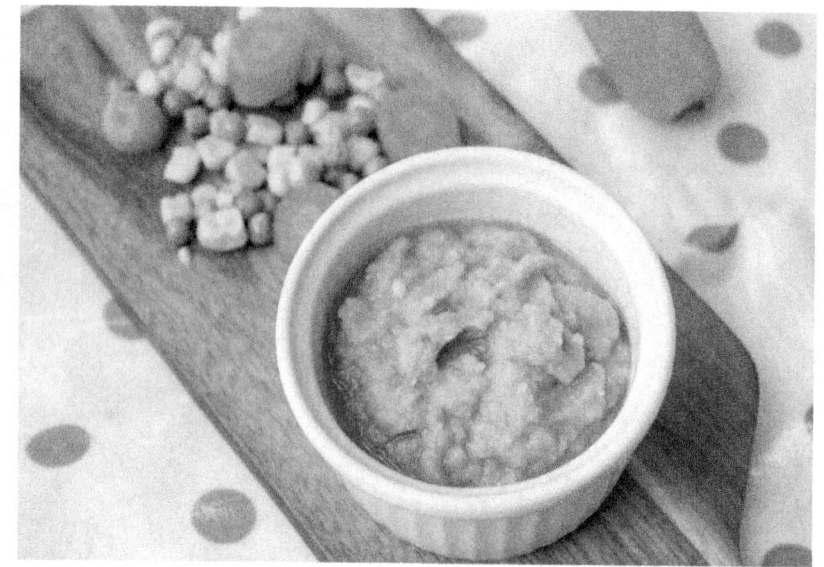

Ingredients

2 teaspoons canola oil	1 garlic clove
1 cup onion	Pepper
4 cups chicken broth	Dash ground nutmeg
1-1/2 cup potatoes	3 cups thinly sliced carrots
1/2 teaspoon sugar	2/3 cup celery

Instructions

1. Cook carrots, ginger, celery, potatoes, garlic, and sugar in oil in a Dutch oven or soup kettle over medium heat for 5 minutes. Bring the broth, pepper, and nutmeg to a simmer, and then add. Reduce the heat, cover, and simmer the vegetables for 30 to 40 minutes or until soft.

2. Cool to average temperatures after being removed from the heat. In a food processor or blender, puree in batches. Heat the kettle thoroughly once more.

Nutrition Facts   Calories: 140 calories, Proteins: 9g, Carbs: 12g, Fat: 9g

Chapter 10: Tips For Dining Out

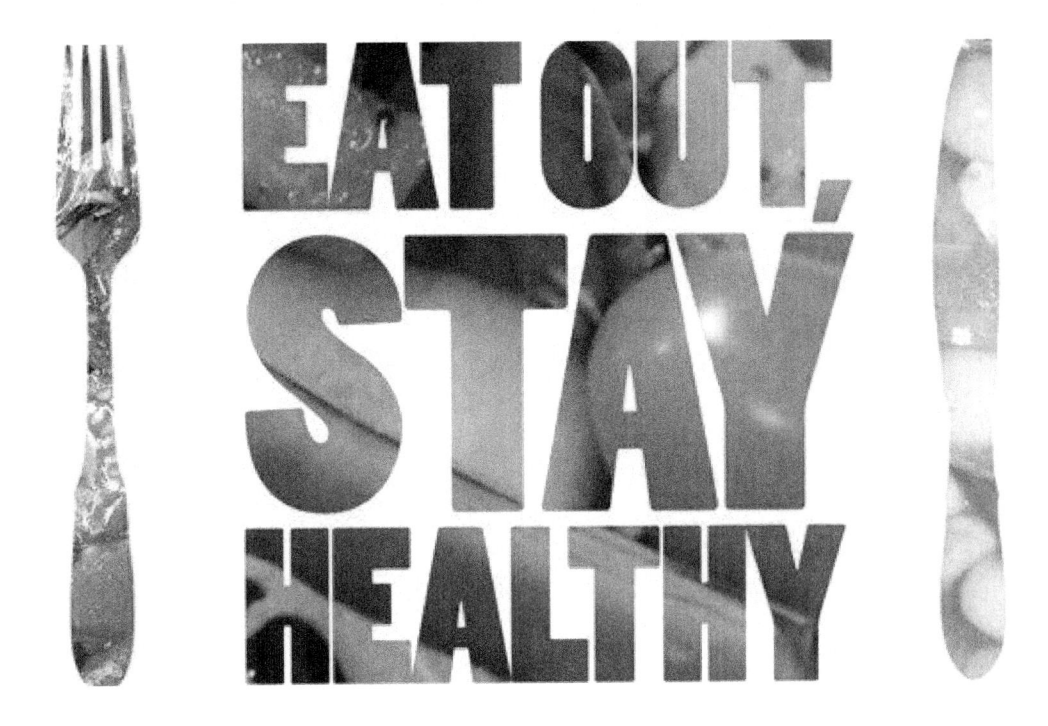

It is not true that you will never be able to eat at any of your favorite restaurants again just because you have had or are undergoing bariatric surgery. Occasionally, we all need a vacation from the task of preparing meals. You have to make informed decisions to provide the body with the nutrition it needs to function properly. Continue reading for useful advice that might alleviate some of officiated with dining at a restaurant.

Researching the restaurant's menu is the most critical thing you can do before going there. Find some foods that you are interested in eating but also fit within the parameters of a healthy diet that you need to adhere to reach the weight reduction target you have set for yourself. If you think about what you will do in advance, you will be better able to resist temptation when hunger strikes. You may be amazed at how amenable certain eateries are to grant your demands if you try them.

- Look for baking, broiling, roasting, grilling, sautéing, or steaming foods.
- Instead of choosing beef or sausage as your protein source, choose leaner options such as chicken breast, shrimp, fish, turkey, mussels, scallops, & Tofu, and be sure to consume your protein first.

- Steer clear of the things on the menu that are fried, crispy, battered, tempura, creamy, or served in a cream sauce or alfredo.
- Don't bother with the bread basket; it's just a waste of calories that won't do anything for you.
- Request healthier alternatives for your sides, such as roasted vegetables, a side salad, or perhaps fruit, instead of high-carbohydrate and high-fat options like french fries, potato chips, onion rings, etc.
- To add taste and moisture to your dish without increasing the calories and salt it contains, ask for dressings, sauces, gravy, butter or sour cream on the side. You may also ask for lime or lemon wedges.
- Do not be in a hurry; instead, eat leisurely, relish each meal, and enjoy the companionship of those around you while you do so.
- Choose soups based on broth rather than creamy soups and vinaigrette dressings rather than creamy dressings.
- Most restaurants provide mostly fried appetizers or heavy calories, but this is rarely the case and depends on the establishment. It is possible that ordering a more nutritious appetizer, which would often be smaller than the main course, will be the superior decision.
- Request that the waiter provides a takeout box together with your entrée. It will allow you to save the other half of your meal for a later time or share an entrée with another person.

10.1: When will you be able to begin eating out?

After bariatric surgery, each individual will go through the eating stages at their own pace. Following gastric sleeve surgery, patients can often only take full liquids for the first two (2) weeks after the procedure. It's possible that between weeks 3 and 4 of the gastric sleeve diet, you'll move to eat soft foods. The process continues with the consumption of solid meals.

After six weeks, it is OK to begin reintroducing solid meals into the diet. Depending on their tolerance level following surgery, it may take up to eight weeks or even longer for some people to return to a regular eating schedule. After gastric sleeve surgery, you may start going to restaurants after reaching the point where you can once again consume solid meals without discomfort. Despite this, portion control is still very important. Eat mindfully at places that are suitable for those with bariatric needs.

10.2: What Food Should One Eat?

Your diet after bariatric surgery is designed to accomplish a very specific goal. It is essential for both healing and continued weight management to adhere to the appropriate dietary requirements. By adhering to the food list with your gastric sleeve, you can consume well-rounded meals high in nutrients while controlling the number of calories you take.

To achieve their recommended daily protein consumption, patients with bariatric surgery need to eat less at each meal. It's advisable to avoid some meals, such as those high in fat or difficult to digest. They are encouraged to consume a well-rounded diet with all the required proteins, vital fatty acids, and fiber. Patients should put a strong emphasis on eating meals that are rich in protein. Ones that are high in nutrients should be consumed rather than meals that are high in calories. You may also find that bariatric vitamins & bariatric protein meal replacement drinks help ensure you continue getting enough nutrition and achieving your daily nutrient objectives.

10.3: Take Control when Selecting Beverage

After bariatric surgery, the ideal beverages to consume are those that do not contain sugar, like water. Try to stay away from consuming your calories by drinking beverages such as alcoholic beverages, soft drinks, juices, and sports drinks. Sugary drinks contain many calories and very little nourishment that the body needs.

After bariatric surgery, patients should usually abstain from caffeine for a certain time. Choose decaffeinated drinks if you want to consume coffee while you wait for additional instructions from your healthcare practitioner. Eating low-fat milk, non-dairy milk substitutes, and protein shakes OK. Consuming carbonated beverages after gastric sleeve surgery is not suggested until at least three months after the procedure. Consuming carbonated drinks before the stomach is ready may have gastrointestinal distress, nausea, and gas due to drinking them. If you consume both food and fluids at the same time, you may notice that you have additional adverse effects. It is advised that liquids be consumed between meals instead of with meals. Wait at least half an hour after finishing a meal before having anything to drink.

10.4: Better Choices From Different Restaurants

Here are some places with excellent options from several categories

Japanese Cuisine - Seaweed salad, Sashimi, edamame, miso soup, Ceviche, tuna tartar, the Naruto sushi roll (which substitutes thinly sliced cucumber for rice), and steamed shrimp dumplings are among examples of Japanese cuisine.

Italian Cuisine – options include grilled chicken, shrimp, salmon salads, chicken cacciatore, chef salads, grilled vegetables, wilted spinach with garlic, sautéed Swiss chard, and roasted or broiled chicken or fish.

Chinese Cuisine – Hot and sour soup, Egg drop soup, egg foo young, steamed vegetables with Tofu, chicken or shrimp, chicken & broccoli, chicken and snow peas, moo goo gai pan, and steamed vegetables are all examples of Chinese cuisine. Steamed or sautéed veggies and meats may be found in "healthy" sections of certain Chinese restaurants. Since sauces are heavy in sugar and salt, request them on the side.

Mexican Cuisine – Chicken tortilla soup, Ceviche, seafood soup, taco salad, churrasco, black beans, burrito bowls even without rice, salsa, Pescado veracruzano, chicken or shrimp mainly based without the tortilla, and siete mares are all examples of Mexican cuisine.

Greek and Mediterranean Cuisine - includes hummus and vegetables, chicken kabobs, a mezze buffet, chicken shawarma, a Greek salad, lentil soup, a tahini salad, baba through, a red cabbage salad, an Israeli salad, and tabbouleh.

Breakfast - options include Greek yogurt parfaits, poached eggs, hard-boiled eggs, egg whites, Canadian bacon, fruit cups, fruit cups, vegetarian omelets, eggs Florentine, veggie omelets, oats with fruit, and turkey bacon and sausage.

Finally, be aware of how people feel after eating. Do you feel content, assured, and in charge? Or maybe crammed, uneasy, and guilty? You will feel more certain that you are in charge and the food does not rule you the more often you go out to eat & have a satisfying experience. Following surgery, you don't have to completely avoid eating out and may still enjoy social gatherings without feeling out of control.

10.5: Extra Tips

Make sure of your partner's likes when ordering since they will get the leftovers.

If you and your spouse or friend are going out to eat, Sarah, who has a gastric sleeve, shared this excellent advice. Because you won't be able to eat a full-sized meal at a restaurant after having weight reduction surgery, you should offer it to someone else if you don't want any food to go to waste. We are not suggesting that you should order to satisfy others and not please yourself, but it is comforting to know that someone can assist you in clearing your plate.

Before you go, make sure you read the menu.

Most restaurants now provide downloadable menus online, so you may plan ahead of time for what the healthiest choice for you is going to be. If, after reading the menu, you can still not discover a meal that is good for your post-bariatric lifestyle, then you might recommend another restaurant that offers a wider variety of dishes appropriate for your diet. You might also take advantage of the live nutritionist help available on our app around the clock. You might offer them the menu and your list of food dos and don'ts and then inquire about what they believe to be the most suitable option.

Request what is known as a "child portion."

Another piece of advice from Sarah, who underwent the gastric sleeve procedure. Do not be hesitant to ask for child-sized dishes or servings on the smaller side. It does not imply that you are required to order from the children's menu, but if you want to dine at one of the many restaurants that provide lower-sized meals, even if they do not publicize the fact, ask!

Tapas!

It would seem that tapas is a favorite among bariatric patients, regardless of whether they have had the band, the sleeve, or the bypass! The wonderful thing about ordering tapas is that you are not required to specify any particular dietary needs or restrictions. Every dish is on the smaller side and meant to be shared. It is a wonderful alternative to consider if you do not want to inform individuals about your surgical procedure.

Tell People.

We know that weight reduction surgery may be a sensitive topic, so many patients only discuss it with a select group of close friends and family members. Nevertheless, if you can discuss your procedure with others, go ahead! When you go out to eat, you won't have to deal with the awkward situation of others asking you why you aren't eating much or taking so long to finish your meal. It is impossible to compete against having the support of those around you.

Conclusion

Surgical procedures can reduce the size of a patient's stomach and alter how their bodies process the food they consume. Patients will undoubtedly consume fewer foods, and their bodies will not be able to fully absorb the caloric value of the food that they do consume. However, maintaining a healthy diet is still vital after weight loss surgery. Not attentive patients could halt their weight loss by making poor food choices or failing to adhere to the 90-30-10 rule.

Unless they are diligent, they could even experience weight gain. Even after the patient has reached their target weight, they will still have to adhere to a healthy diet and pay close attention to the foods they consume. Suppose the patient returns to their former habits, such as munching, drinking beverages high in calories, eating meals rich in sugar and fat, and not exercising every day. In that case, their success in losing weight may only persist for 18 months, and they may even face a rebound. The foundation of a healthy lifestyle is proper nutrition, achieved through eating well-balanced meals. After having bariatric surgery, you must adjust how you usually eat. After surgery, the patient's diet will continue through a predetermined plan to reduce the risk of lactose intolerance and other nutrition-related issues.

The diet development is meant to make it easier for you to heal. When you first wake up after surgery, your primary objective will be to consume enough liquid and protein through a liquid-based diet to satisfy your requirements. Your nutritional requirements for long-term health will be better met as time passes, and you can eat a wider variety, including whole foods that are naturally low in sugar and saturated fat. This will allow you to better satisfy your nutritional demands. During the first four days after having, you will need to adjust your eating routine to reduce or eliminate feelings of nausea and vomiting and jumpstart losing weight. You must cultivate healthy eating habits to maintain a good BMI and avoid gaining weight. To get the best out of the food you eat while consuming the fewest calories possible, you must be conscious of the maximum amount of food you can consume in one sitting and choose nutritious options. Changing physical activity to a regular part of your schedule is essential to avoid gaining weight again.

Invite to Review Book

I am grateful that you took the time to read my book. I hope that you found it to be both pleasant and educational. As an author, I place a high value on the comments and suggestions made by my readers, and I would be very interested in hearing your opinions regarding the book.

If you get a chance, I'd appreciate it if you could leave a review on the platform of your choice whenever you get a chance. Your review has the potential to assist other readers in locating the book in question and making an educated choice regarding whether or not to read it.

I appreciate any comments, recommendations, or criticisms you may have, and I will do my best to incorporate them into future revisions. I am grateful you took the time to read my book, and I look forward to hearing from you soon.

With warmest regards,

Angela Ramsey

Printed in Great Britain
by Amazon